Clean Eating Cookbook

The All-in-1 Healthy Eating Guide – 153 Quick & Easy Recipes, A Weekly Shopping List & More!

by Olivia Rogers

Copyright © 2017 By Olivia Rogers
All rights reserved. No part of this book may be reproduced in any form without permission in writing from the author. No part of this publication may be reproduced or transmitted in any form or by any means, mechanic, electronic, photocopying, recording, by any storage or retrieval system, or transmitted by email without the permission in writing from the author and publisher.
For information regarding permissions write to author at
Olivia@TheMenuAtHome.com
Reviewers may quote brief passages in review.

Please note that credit for the images used in this book go to the respective owners. You can view this at: TheMenuAtHome.com/image-list

Olivia Rogers
TheMenuAtHome.com

Table of Contents

Who is this book for? 10
What will this book teach you? 10
Introduction 11
Chapter 1: The Secret to A Slim Body 13
Chapter 2: What are Thermogenic Foods? 14
Chapter 3: Incredible Benefits of Thermogenic Foods 15
Chapter 4: Thermogenic Superfoods 16
Chapter 5: Thermogenic Lean Protein Foods 18
Chapter 6: Thermogenic Vegetarian Protein Foods 19
Chapter 7: Thermogenic Fiber Rich Foods 20
Chapter 8: Thermogenic Seeds and Nuts 22
Chapter 9: Thermogenic Spices 23
Chapter 10: Healthy Veggies and Fruits 25
Chapter 11: Healthy Proteins 30
Chapter 12: Healthy Drinks 33
Chapter 13: Healthy Whole Grains 34
Chapter 14: Healthy Dairy 35
Chapter 15: Recipe Meals 36
1. Herbal Arugula Soup 36
2. Broccoli Omelet with Toast 37
3. Lettuce and Chicken Salad 38
4. Grapefruit Avocado and Salmon Salad 39
5. Mushrooms with Vegetable Stuffing 40
6. Crispy and Cheesy Zucchini Rings 41
7. Grapefruit and Kale Salad 42

8. Chocolate Chip Pumpkin Bread _____ 43
9. Radish and Cucumber Fry with Noodles_____ 44
10. Spicy Green Tea _____ 45
11. Celery Root and Apple Salad_____ 46
12. Berry Smoothie _____ 47
13. Classic Carrot-Ginger Soup_____ 48
14. Oats and Dark Chocolate Clusters _____ 49
15. Avocado Tomato and Lettuce Sandwich_____ 50
16. Pineapple Salsa and Pan-Grilled Salmon _____ 50
17. Cheesy Pear_____ 51
18. Citrus and Ginger Salad_____ 52
19. Almond French Toast_____ 53
20. Minty Ice Tea _____ 54
21. Brown Lentil Soup _____ 55
22. Duck-Confit and Blood Orange Salad _____ 56
23. Pan-Fried Pine Nuts and Brussels Sprouts _____ 57
24. Chocolate-Milk Shake _____ 58
25. Roasted Quinoa with Corn _____ 58
26. Avocado & Egg Toast_____ 59
27. Breakfast Burrito_____ 60
28. Banana Carrot Muffins_____ 61
29. Ham & Cheese Quinoa Bites_____ 62
30. Cranberry Quinoa Muffins_____ 63
31. Pumpkin Oatmeal _____ 65
32. Avocado Wraps _____ 66
33. Spinach & Egg Pizza_____ 67
34. Carrot & Lentil Soup _____ 68

35. Tuna Stuffed Summer Squash _____ 69
36. Butternut Squash Salad _____ 70
37. Tomato Chorizo Salad _____ 71
38. Chicken Breasts Stuffed with Feta & Sundried Tomatoes __ 72
39. Salmon on A Bed of Spinach, Pears & Blue Cheese _____ 73
40. Chicken Walnut Berry Salad _____ 74
41. Lemon Pepper Tuna on A Bed of Veggie Couscous _____ 75
42. Maple Pecan Pork Chops _____ 77
43. Healthy Whole Wheat and Oats Pumpkin Pancakes _____ 78
44. Low-Fat and Healthy Buttermilk Waffles _____ 79
45. Coconut Chocolate Energy Truffle Recipe _____ 80
46. Deep Dark Chocolate Layer Cake _____ 82
47. Low Fat Strawberry Cheesecake _____ 83
48. Creamy Cheese Chocolate Chip Cookies _____ 84
49. Low-Cal, Low-Fat Mashed Potatoes with Crispy Golden Chicken _____ 86
50. Crispy Golden Chicken _____ 87
51. Chicken Breasts Stuffed with Pimiento Cheese _____ 88
52. Black Bean and Quinoa Burgers _____ 89
53. Creamy Tarragon Chicken Salad _____ 90
54. Fish and Chips with Tartar Sauce _____ 91
55. Roasted Red Pepper, Hummus, Avocado & Feta Sandwich _ 93
56. Mom's Easy Healthy Baked Beans _____ 94
57. Quick Fall Minestrone _____ 95
58. Healthier World's Best Lasagna _____ 96
59. Low-Calorie Cauliflower Crust Pizza (Gluten Free) _____ 98
60. Squash and Tomato Casserole _____ 99

61. Mom's Creamy Chicken and Broccoli Casserole _____ 101
62. Ground Beef and Texas Bean Enchiladas_____ 102
63. Low Salt, Low Fat Turkey Sloppy Joes _____ 103
64. Sweet Potato Hash Browns_____ 104
65. Curried Butternut Squash Bisque _____ 105
66. Asparagus and Chicken Noodle Casserole _____ 106
67. Harvest Port and Butternut Squash Stew_____ 107
68. Halibut and Corn Chowder _____ 108
69. Pork Kebabs with Honey _____ 109
70. Four Bean Salad _____ 110
71. Crock Pot Jambalaya _____ 111
72. Sweet Potato Fish Cakes_____ 112
73. Sweet Potato Fritters_____ 113
74. Brown Sugar Barbecue Chicken _____ 114
75. Chicken and Sweetcorn Macaroni _____ 114
76. Confetti Spaghetti Salad_____ 115
77. Beef and Curry Pasta _____ 116
78. Tandoori Chicken _____ 117
79. Spiced Salmon with Chili Sauce_____ 118
80. Slow Cooked Stuffed Gammon _____ 119
81. Potato and Pork Bake_____ 120
82. Summer Cabbage Soup with Sausages _____ 121
83. Teriyaki Fried Rice with Chicken _____ 121
84. Sea Bass with Orange and Honey_____ 122
85. Slow Cooker Breakfast Casserole _____ 123
86. Slow Cooker Jambalaya_____ 124
87. Spaghetti Bolognaise_____ 125

88. Beef and Vegetable Parmesan _____ 126
89. Fried Green Tomatoes _____ 127
90. Mushroom and Cabbage Stroganoff _____ 128
91. Beef and Portobello Stroganoff _____ 129
92. Chili Con Carne _____ 130
93. Baked Sweet Potatoes with Sour Cream _____ 131
94. Breakfast Barley with Sunflower Seeds and Banana _____ 132
95. Curried Egg Salad Sandwich _____ 133
96. Salmon Noodle Bowl _____ 134
97. Chicken Chilaquiles and Black Bean _____ 135
98. Pan-grilled Salmon with Pineapple Salsa _____ 136
99. Italian Garbanzo Salad _____ 137
100. Greek Yogurt Fruit Parfait _____ 138
101. Toasted Hazelnut, Raw Kale and Grapefruit Salad _____ 139
102. Creamy Avocado Cups _____ 140
103. Oat Clusters & Dark Chocolate _____ 141
104. Spiced Green Tea Smoothie _____ 142
105. Chocolate-Dipped Banana Bites _____ 143
106. Banana & Almond Butter Toast _____ 144
107. Honey Grapefruit with Banana _____ 144
108. Broccoli and Feta Omelet with Toast _____ 145
109. White Bean & Herb Hummus with Crudites _____ 146
110. BBQ Turkey Burgers _____ 147
111. Middle Eastern Rice Salad _____ 148
112. Energy-stimulating Quinoa _____ 149
113. Avocado Whip _____ 150
114. Crisp Chickpea Slaw _____ 151

115. Spicy Southwestern Black Bean Chili _____ 152
116. Avocado Peach Salad _____ 153
117. Red-Lentil Hummus Sandwich _____ 154
118. Banana Nut Oatmeal _____ 155
119. Greek Lentil Soup with Toasted Pita _____ 156
120. Sunflower Lentil Spread _____ 157
121. Vegan Caprese Salad _____ 158
122. Spiced Banana-Almond Smoothie _____ 159
123. Rice and Egg Salad-to-Go _____ 160
124. All-American Chili _____ 161
125. Strawberry Cauliflower Salad Delight _____ 162
126. Creamy Cauliflower Salad with Ranch _____ 163
127. Salad made with Shredded Brussels Sprouts _____ 164
128. Brussels Sprouts with Chili Flakes and Pumpkin Seeds Topping _____ 165
129. Raw Pesto Pasta with Pine Nuts and Carrots _____ 165
130. Tangy Kale Pesto _____ 166
131. Kelp Noodles with Pesto Pasta _____ 167
132. Spinach Basil Pesto with Raw Noodles _____ 168
133. Ravioli Made with Beets and Served with Pesto Oil _____ 169
134. Pine Nuts Cheese _____ 170
135. Avocado Pesto with Parsley _____ 171
136. Kale and Avocado Salad with Raw Black Olives _____ 172
137. Walnut, Celery and Apple Salad with Kale _____ 173
138. Mango Salad with Peaches and Lemon _____ 174
139. Grapes and Melon Salad _____ 174
140. Raw Tuna Salad Recipe _____ 175

141. Basil and Cucumber Salad _____ 176
142. Apple and Apricot Salad with Ginger Dressing and Walnuts _____ 177
143. Red Cabbage Salad _____ 177
144. Sugar Snap Pea Salad _____ 178
145. Crunchy Green Apple and Red Cabbage Salad _____ 179
146. Rainbow Salad with Coconut Oil _____ 180
147. Fiesta Carrot Salad _____ 181
148. Walnut Salad with Guacamole Dressing _____ 181
149. Raw Vegan Version of Waldorf Salad _____ 182
150. Costa Rican Tomato Salad with Lime _____ 183
151. Watermelon and Peach Salad with Lime _____ 184
152. Orange Salad with Avocado and Black Olives _____ 185
153. Strawberry and Spinach Salad _____ 186
Final Words _____ 187
Disclaimer _____ 188

Who is this book for?

They who are suffering from overweight know the feeling how it ruins every aspect of their life and makes a huge negative impact on their career, relationships, satisfaction and self-esteem. You might have a buzzing social life, little time to cook or a fascination for delicious but high-calorie food and weighed down with overweight but don't know or have time to get your dream shape without taking away entire food groups, creepy supplements or starvation.

Well, if dropping weight and stay healthy is your aim and you want to get the result without giving much effort and time, this book can lend you a hand to start the ball rolling on a path of small steps and you may be amazed to see how it can ensure a considerable weight loss within a short period of time and, most importantly, quite effortlessly. Without starving yourself, eating at unusual times of the day only or throwing out your social life, you'd be able to have the satisfaction that comes from knowing that you are in control of your life.

This book will greatly benefit health conscious people who are also food lovers and yet want to stay fit and live a long life. Also, the recipes included in this book are for people who want or need to lose weight while still being able to have comfort foods. A common-sense approach to healthy eating by focusing on what you can eat, and not on what you have to give up, will help you get results without feeling deprived. Once you know how many calories to consume, you can enjoy your meals with low calorie yet exceptionally tasty versions of your favorite foods, with the entire family.

What will this book teach you?

The key to accomplishing and continuing to remain healthy isn't about dietary changes on a short-term basis. It's about a way of life that comprises eating well, daily physical exercise, and balancing the number of calories you consume with the number of calories your body uses. In this book, you can find:

- Great tasting recipes that are healthy too
- All recipes assessed by registered nutritionists
- Offers comfort foods that are satisfying for the whole family
- Dieting without having to give up some of your favorite foods
- Learn to eat sensibly and keep the weight off
- Low-calorie editions of hearty foods

Introduction

Comfort foods in this cookbook offer the finest of both worlds. You'll get great tasting foods that are low in calories and will help in weight loss. All of the recipes are evaluated by dieticians and are the sort of foods that your whole family will relish. Home cooking presents a lot of options and full control over what you're eating. You would be amazed what little alterations can make some of your favourite foods healthier. Some of the recipes you will find are:

- Pizza
- Lasagna
- Strawberry Cheesecake
- Fried Chicken tenders
- Pumpkin Pancakes
- Mashed Potatoes
- Chocolate truffle

Obesity is one of the major health problems in most of the developed countries around the world. Latest WHO statics reveal that over 600 million populations suffer from this unhealthy condition. The major reason of being overweight is sedentary lifestyle and consumption of unhealthy food. With modern hectic life, people hardly find any time for exercise and outdoor activities. Including thermogenic food proves an effective method to burn extra calories. Making these foods a regular part of your meal melts stubborn body fats.

The present book will also give you some of the best fat-blasting thermogenic foods and how they help to melt calories effectively just by consuming them. A key basis for any healthy diet is self-control that means having only as much food as your body requires. Instead of getting overfed, you should feel fulfilled at the end of a meal. Self-control is also about balance. We all need a balance of fiber, fat, protein, carbohydrates, minerals and vitamins to maintain a healthy body. It means eating less of the insalubrious food (saturated fat, refined sugar etc.) and replacing it with the healthy stuff (vegetables, fresh fruit, lean protein etc.).

It's true that some foods have a very high thermogenic effect that burn calories while you chomp. Some other foods contain compounds and nutrients that add fuel to your metabolic fire that trim down your hunger and appetite significantly thus do away with the key factor that most people fail with usual weight loss methods. If you don't know how to work these calorie-burning ingredients into your everyday menu, start with the recipes mentioned in this book. They all incorporate at least one weight-loss superfood, and, the best part is, they can be prepared in thirty minutes or less!

When you are just starting out, healthy eating can seem like an impossibly difficult task. You might think choosing to eat healthy means choosing to give up flavor and enjoyment. But this is a myth spread by those who don't know how to eat healthy!

In reality, healthy food is usually more flavorful and delicious than unhealthy food. There are so many amazing (and healthy) ingredients out there that you'll never get bored with your new, healthy lifestyle. To help get you started, this book will give you irresistibly yummy recipes that will make you wonder why anyone ever thought healthy eating couldn't taste good.

The generally held belief that our supermarkets are stuffed with unhealthy, canned foods imported from God-knows-where is absolutely misleading. This book proves, without an iota of doubt that there are plenty of foods and other related edible products in our supermarkets that are indeed healthy and highly recommendable for everyone's consumption. Highlighted in this book are some great, rare finds that include foods, fruits, vegetables and drinks of different kinds. The criteria for selecting the ones included in this book are based on five essential factors:

- They contain life-enriching nutrients and vitamins that are required in day-to-day metabolic activities.
- They contain little calories and hence cannot cause fattening in human bodies.
- They are naturally or organically made: but when they required some additives, in case of some desserts, very limited quantities of food additives were used.
- They are available in supermarkets across the globe; you can find these foods, drinks, vegetables and fruits near you.
- They are affordable and a little quantity of them can produce significant, healthy results in your body.

So, next time you walk into a supermarket, have it in your mind that the place actually holds some great finds you can buy to improve your health, maintain your weight and live a long life. You don't have to bother yourself about drawing up the appropriate healthy shopping list anymore; we have done the hard job for you by researching at supermarkets which foods, drinks, proteins, fruits and vegetables will possibly improve your health and that of your loved ones. It is an effort that took us some years before we finally settled on these recipes that will surely have some positive impacts on your health.

Try each of the recipes out and don't be afraid to experiment and modify the recipes. Get creative and have fun! In this book, you will find some scrumptious recipes for the whole month, so you don't have to worry about what to put on your menu for the next days. Bon Appetite!

Chapter 1: The Secret to A Slim Body

Who does not love to have a well-toned body with a flat belly? Those superfluous layers of fat around the waistline and hips spoil the entire look of your sleek outfit. Not to forget the armpits sagging under stubborn fat deposits and those bulging thighs that refrain you from wearing your favorite bikini. You often look back on how slim you were few years ago and looked amazing in that aqua green bikini. Most of us wonder how we have gradually started putting on weight over these years. Do you wish to get back in your perfect figure and flaunt your curves? Do you simply want to look sizzling in a bikini over the beach side and leave your friends awestruck? We are going to make all this possible for you now.

The secret to burning stubborn body fat

The good news is now you can melt all those extra pounds accumulated over the long run. Food is one of the major factors influencing and controlling body weight. What you eat determines your body weight and body mass index. Those excess fats can be trimmed by making slight alterations to your diet. A slim body starts from the kitchen rather than from the gym. So, read on to find how thermogenic food can help you get rid of those flabby unwanted fat and bring a new transformation within you.

Read This FIRST - 100% FREE BONUS

FOR A LIMITED TIME ONLY – Get Olivia's best-selling book *"The #1 Cookbook: Over 170+ of the Most Popular Recipes Across 7 Different Cuisines!"* absolutely FREE!

Readers have absolutely loved this book because of the wide variety of recipes. It is highly recommended you check these recipes out and see what you can add to your home menu!

Once again, as a big thank-you for downloading this book, I'd like to offer it to you *100% FREE for a LIMITED TIME ONLY!*

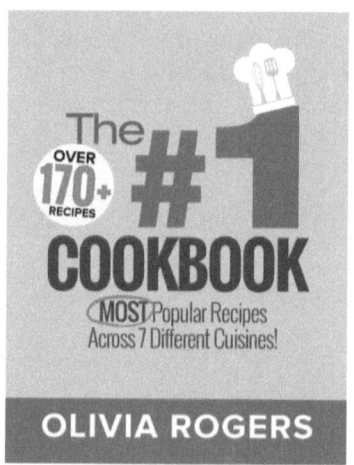

Get your free copy at:

TheMenuAtHome.com/Bonus

Chapter 2: What are Thermogenic Foods?

The best method to burn fat from the comfort of home is to include thermogenic food in regular diet. This form of diet is proven one of the most effective weight loss methods. Just eat these wonderful fat blasting foods to cut down excess pounds. Adoption of thermogenic diet stokes metabolic rate, doubles the chances of losing calories, trims waistline and melts stubborn fat deposits.

So, what are thermogenic foods?

Our body utilizes energy and burns calories for digesting food. Foods that utilize the body's maximum energy for proper digestion are referred to as thermogenic foods. These foods are known to produce high thermogenic effect within the body. Thermogenic effect, also referred to as thermogenesis, enhances the body's metabolic rate and burns extra calories when the food is being digested.

Thermogenic foods are best fat blasting diets. They produce thermogenesis, increase the metabolic rate, utilize energy from the body to burn calories and digest the ingested food. During metabolic rate, the fat deposits of the body are burnt to produce heat within the body. Extra calories and deposited fats are effectively burnt during this entire process. Some of the best thermogenic foods are lean proteins and food with high contents of fiber, protein, vitamins, nutrients, minerals, antioxidants and essential vegetable fats.

Why are thermogenic foods the ultimate fat melting diets?

Thermogenic foods are packed with certain stimulants for higher thermogenesis. The reaction of these stimulants burn fat and produces body heat thus accelerating the body's metabolic rate. The stimulants accelerate the rate of heart beat and metabolic rate. Some of the powerful stimulants present in thermogenic food include caffeine, capsaicin and catechins.

Moderate doses of caffeine have proven effective in burning fat deposits. Capsaicin is a compound present in hot peppers. Studies prove that the compound increases the process of thermogenesis. Catechins are known to stimulate thermogenesis and enhance fat oxidation. Foods containing these stimulants increases body heat and melt fat for an effective weight loss.

Chapter 3: Incredible Benefits of Thermogenic Foods

Now that the importance of adopting fat burning food is known, let us in detail explore some of the top most food that comes under this category. Lean proteins, green tea, certain spices and vegetable oils, green leafy vegetables and fiber rich foods all contribute to healthy weight loss straight away from your kitchen.

The present book reveals fat-blasting foods you wish you knew to melt fat deposits and cut down your waistline. Some of the healthiest and nutritional dense food that stokes the metabolic process is mentioned here. The book also covers the importance of including aromatic spices for effective weight loss.

Thermogenic food for effective calorie burning

Here are seven incredible benefits of adapting thermogenic foods to your regular meal plan

1. Enhances the metabolic rate
2. Utilizes maximum energy of the body during digestion
3. Burns extra calories for effective weight loss
4. Doubles the chances of losing weight
5. Decreases the chances of obesity and other illness related to over weight
6. Adds low calorie, nutritional dense food to meal plan
7. Provides a feeling of fullness with limited calorie consumption

Chapter 4: Thermogenic Superfoods

Superfoods are nutritional powerhouses packed with high nutritional content, essential vitamins, minerals, antioxidants and fibers. Inclusion of these super healthy foods help meet the body's nutritional requirement, produce thermogenic effect, melt extra calories, prevents several diseases such as cancer, cardiac problems, diabetes and obesity.

Superfoods for super slim body

Indulge in superfoods to get super slim body. Here are some of the top superfoods you need to add to your regular meal.

- **Quinoa**

    Small seeds with mighty benefits, quinoas are most popular superfood worldwide. They are power packs of proteins, minerals and fibers. This unique gluten-free power food comes with nine amino acids essential for nourishment of a healthy body and enhances weight loss. A bowl of warm quinoa tossed with rich greens makes a perfect start to a great day.

- **Green tea**

    Green tea is regarded as one of the best ingredients to lose stubborn fats. The presence of powerful antioxidant called epigallocatechin gallate (EGCG) is known to attribute to its high thermogenic property. Green tea extracts act as excellent metabolism boosters. This fat melting ingredient filled with phytonutrients and antioxidants is known to stoke metabolic activity as high as four percent within a time frame of 24 hours.

- **Tomatoes**

    Juicy tomatoes are high source of antioxidants. Though technically a fruit, tomatoes are considered as vegetables. Considered best among weight loss food, ripe tomatoes make up to 95% of water content with the remaining 5% being insoluble fiber and carbohydrate.

- **Grapefruit**

    This citrus fruit contains fewer calories and is loaded with vitamin C, essential nutrients and antioxidants. It is proven to increase the metabolic rate, detoxify the entire body and ensure a glowing complexion. Grapefruit contains a component called pectin that lowers blood cholesterol. Regular consumption of grapefruit helps to keep a check on unwanted fat deposits for a flatter belly.

- **Mushrooms**

    Mushrooms are delicious food with weight loss properties. Basically, from the fungus family, mushrooms are rich sources of powerful antioxidants and phytonutrients. Research proves that consumption of mushrooms regulates blood glucose level. Besides adding flavor to food, mushrooms protects against damage of tissues.

- **Kale**

    This leafy green vegetable is low in calories and high in thermogenic properties. Its high fiber content gives a feeling of fullness keeping away from calorie bombs. Kale is considered 'super' among superfood with its rich fiber content, vitamin C, K and A as well as high phytonutrients.

- **Berries**

Berries are powerhouses of wonderful phytonutrients, antioxidants and weigh losing compounds. These juicy fruits are known to protect the entire system from illness, prevent intestinal disorders, type2 diabetes and cancer risks.

Chapter 5: Thermogenic Lean Protein Foods

Lean proteins are filled with essential macronutrients that that help repair body tissues and muscles. Protein rich food requires high energy for digestion and metabolism thus burning more calories during this process. Lean proteins are low in fat and rich in essential amino acids that help develop lean muscles and lose fat. It is important to include the right amount of protein in your diet to increase metabolic rate, melt fat and reduce weight.

Proteins for lean toned body

Here are some of the best lean proteins to go for. Kick start your day by adding considerable amount of these proteins for a healthy feeling.

- **Egg whites**

    Egg whites are considered good sources of lean proteins. The white potion of egg has fewer calories and high proteins when compared to its yellow yolk portion. Proteins dramatically enhance the metabolic rate by 3 percent melting more fat. Just swap the yolk portion with enough whites to make a delicious low-calorie meal. Studies reveal that people who consumed egg whites burnt stomach fat more effectively.

- **Fish**

    Fish comes with satisfying flavor and health benefits. Tuna, salmons, sardines and other fatty fishes are considered rich sources of omega-3 fatty acids, protein, potassium, calcium and other essential nutrients for a healthy body. The essential fats found in fish are useful to burn calories, reduce bad cholesterol levels and prevent blood from easy clotting reducing risks of heart attacks.

- **Chicken breast**

    Lean proteins in chicken breasts make a full meal with fewer calories and fats. This means eating few calories and burning more of it. Lean proteins also help to gain ideal body mass and increase energy expenditure of the body for effective weight loss.

Chapter 6: Thermogenic Vegetarian Protein Foods

Proteins are also known as the building blocks of the body. They are essential for muscle building and help effective fat loss. Studies prove that protein rich food causes higher thermogenic effect than high fat or high carbohydrate food. Vegetable proteins come with the benefit of high protein content and less fat when compared to non-vegetarian protein versions.

The best low-fat proteins for slim waistline

Munch on these ultimate low-fat vegetarian proteins to meet your daily protein intake and burn your fats easily. Here are some of the best thermogenic vegetarian protein sources to narrow the waistline.

- **Soy**

    Soy is regarded as a complete source of protein. Soy chunks prove an ideal protein substitute for meat. Tofu is regarded as one of the best soy products with loads of proteins and minerals.

- **Green peas**

    Green peas are considered among healthiest food due to their rich protein content and zero percent fat. One cup of green peas contains protein equivalent to a cup of milk. Vegetarians and people intolerant to lactose can meet their protein requirement from green peas.

- **Beans**

    There are varieties of beans to choose from such as black beans, pinto beans, kidney beans, white beans, etc. But they all have one great thing in common, excellent proteins. Beans add the required protein punch in addition to other essential nutrients to your meals and make you easily fill up without indulging in high calories. Beans are considered as one of the cheapest and simplest form of vegetarian proteins. Dry beans can be soaked overnight for easy use.

- **Chick peas**

    Also referred to as garbanzo beans, these protein rich legumes offer high fiber content and low calories. Adding chickpeas to diet increases metabolic rate for effective weight loss. These legumes also contain high potassium content and are low in sodium content.

- **Corn**

    Corns are actually grains that deliver high content of protein with zero fat percentage. Chewing on corns satisfies appetite while literally burning down the calories. They also decrease the risk of cardiovascular and other diseases related to obesity.

- **Mung beans**

    Adding yellow mung beans to the shopping cart is a must for people who aspire to lose weight. Mung beans are high in proteins and low in saturated fat, sodium and cholesterol. With high fullness factor, mung beans are considered ideal food for effective weight loss. Mung beans sprouts offer higher nutritional content.

- **Cottage cheese**

    Low fat cottage cheese is the perfect high protein and low-calorie food to swap with meat. It proves a nutritious low-calorie breakfast or snack. This nutrient dense food helps build lean muscles and maintains healthy teeth and bones.

Chapter 7: Thermogenic Fiber Rich Foods

A healthy digestive track promotes a healthy body. Fiber rich foods are a rich source of both soluble and insoluble fibers that contribute to healthy weight loss. High fiber content food requires higher energy to breakdown thus burning more calories for proper digestion. Soluble fibers absorb bad cholesterols whereas insoluble fibers satisfy appetite with fullness preventing excess calorie consumption. Fibers also add weight to the digested food for smooth digestive functioning and prevent constipation.

Fiber for healthy pipes and effective weight loss

Include these fiber rich foods to add weight to your food for clear bowls and healthy pipes without adding weight to your body.

- **Oats**

    The health benefits of oats are immense. Oatmeal contains soluble and insoluble fibers. The insoluble fibers partly dissolve with water to form gel that absorbs cholesterol related substances from the body. Only bad cholesterol is absorbed without affecting the level of good cholesterol in the bloodstream.

- **Brown rice**

    The high fiber content in brown rice makes the body burn twice the calories when compared to processed food. The insoluble fibers of brown rice give a natural feeling of fullness. This avoids intake of more calories and promote weight loss. The indigestible fiber also helps prevent constipation to maintain a healthy body.

- **Whole grains**

    Consumption of whole grains helps the body to burn 50% more calories than consumption of refined food. Whole grains offer high nutritional density requiring more energy for digestion thus burning your calories naturally. They are reservoirs of rich protein, mineral, fiber, vitamin B and photochemical.

- **Millet**

    This wonderful grain is a boon for vegetarians who are looking to burn calories. Millet is rich in fiber, protein and complex carbohydrate which keeps you full and enhances weight loss naturally. Studies prove that millet contains several nutrients such as vitamin B, magnesium and phytonutrients that increase thermogenic effect.

- **Carrots**

    This colorful vegetable with a natural sweet taste makes it favorite food of people and Bugs Bunny as well. Carrots are packed with high fiber, antioxidants, beta carotene and other vitamins that help to get a perfect bikini besides boosting the immunity system. The best way to eat carrot is in its raw form when all its nutrients remain intact. Make sure to wash them thoroughly to remove any traces of mud and unwanted matter.

- **Cabbage**

    The strong flavor of cabbage imparts delicious flavor to certain dishes. This leafy vegetable is a dietary booster besides providing a considerable source of vitamin C and phytonutrients. Cabbage is considered dieter's best friend. Regular intake of cabbage especially in its raw form is known to give a slim waistline and prevent ageing.

- **Green leafy vegetables**

Green leafy vegetables are extremely nutritious food. From Swiss chard and lettuce to spinach, all of them are packed with high fibrous content and important nutrients that fire up the metabolic rate for a trimmed figure. Leafy vegetables are best eaten sautéed to retain their valuable nutrients which get destroyed if overcooked.

Chapter 8: Thermogenic Seeds and Nuts

Seeds and nuts are loaded with essential oils, fiber, antioxidants and plant based fats that help reduce the bad cholesterol level and melt fatty tissues for natural weight loss. These fat-burning foods are rich in unsaturated fats that reduce the body's saturated fat content. A handful of nuts and seeds everyday maintains a healthy body, healthy heart and promotes weight loss.

Fats for melting body fat

Snack on these thermogenic seeds and nuts to reap the benefits of essential omega-3 fats to melting body fat.

- **Flax seeds**

    These tiny seeds with mighty benefits are exceptional thermogenic food. The goodness of flax seeds excels with its loads of high fibrous content, nutritional value, antioxidants and rich omega-3 fatty acids. The seeds are filled with some of the essential fats that the body is incapable of producing. Intake of flax seeds helps prevent constipation, fight several diseases and most.

- **Coconuts**

    Coconuts are reservoirs of natural vegetable oils which are actually healthy and good for weight loss. Delicious coconut water and coconut meat contains high nutritional content and considered good to maintain an ideal weight. They are packed with essential oils, fiber and nutrients that produce magical effect for a healthy and beautiful body.

- **Chia seeds**

    These tiny nutritious black seeds with low calories list among world's top superfood category. Chia literally means strength. These seeds are loaded with powerful nutrients, antioxidants, rich fiber, magnesium, magnesium and other minerals. They are considered as 'whole grains' and 'gluten free' food. The fiber in chia seeds absorbs water to swell up and fill up the stomach.

- **Sesame seeds**

  Sesame seeds are known to add unique flavor to several dishes. These seeds hold high protein and mineral content. The presence of magnesium, calcium and vitamin E boosts the body's metabolism rate and naturally burns body fat. Its fiber content satisfies appetite and enhances digestion.

- **Hemp seeds**

  Hemp seeds are powerhouse of omega-3 fatty acids that help burn the fat content of the body. These seeds contain high level of iron and magnesium that boosts energy levels. Its potassium content is known to prevent bloating.

- **Almonds**

  Almonds are considered healthiest among fat burning foods. These wonderful nuts are packed with high fiber content that satisfies hunger and promotes weight loss. They are also filled with mono-saturated fats and vitamin E for a healthy heart, hair and skin. Stay trim, healthy and beautiful with almonds.

- **Peanuts**

  Peanuts are considered healthiest among nuts. They are a rich source of mono-saturated fats, folic acid, antioxidants and flavonoids. The natural vegetable oil in these nuts produces thermogenic effect in the body.

Chapter 9: Thermogenic Spices

Spices are flavor boosters that kick metabolism and increase thermogenic effect within the body. Research proves that spices contain anti-inflammatory properties that promote weight loss. These wonderful, aromatic ingredients when used rightly prove the potential to enhance metabolism, aid digestion, promote effective weight management and enhance flavor and quality of food. Herbal drinks and decoctions prepared from spices work magically to melt fat and cut pounds.

Sweet flavors for melting fats

Use these aromatic spices to add flavor to your food and initiate thermogenesis within the body.

- **Cayenne pepper**

    The good thing about adding hot cayenne peppers to food is they heat up your body stoking thermogenic effect to melt those extra calories. Capsaicin is a compound found in peppers that make them hot and impart spiciness to food.

- **Ginger**

    Ginger roots are a reservoir of immense health benefits. They aid digestion, prevent cold and increase immunity. Ginger contains natural anti-inflammatory property that helps to lose weight. Studies prove that the root's thermogenic property speeds the metabolism rate burning some additional fat. Studies suggest that consuming ginger powder dissolved in warm water accelerates thermogenesis for potential weight loss.

- **Black pepper**

    Black peppers add a wonderful flavor and spiciness to food. They are proven to increase the metabolic rate, react with the belly fat and breakdown the fat cells with ease. They also detoxify the body and strengthen immunity against cold. However, it is important to consume these hot spices within limit to prevent gastric problems.

- **Cinnamon**

    This delicious spice is known from ages for its numerous health benefits. The sweet spice is known to regulate blood sugar levels and resist food craving saving from carbs and excess fat. It contains natural essential oils and antioxidants that prevent cancer and regulate insulin level.

- **Cumin**

    Cumin has been used in traditional medicines due to its numerous health benefits. The spice contains a plant chemical known as phytosterols that absorbs cholesterol from the body. Research proves these flavorful seeds kick the metabolic rate and contribute to weight loss.

- **Turmeric**

    Natural antiseptic and antibacterial property of turmeric makes it an integral part of Ayurvedic medicines. Curcumin, a compound found in turmeric produces thermogenic effect in the body for effective fat loss. Angiogenesis property of turmeric prevents the formation of fat cells thus restricting the growth of fat tissues.

- **Cardamom**

    The sweet-smelling spice cardamom increases fat metabolism within the body. The spice aids digestion and prevents digestive ailments. Sipping cardamom tea increases the body's fat burning ability, fights radicals and detoxifies the entire system.

- **Fennel**

    Fennel seeds impart a sweet and mild flavor to dishes. These tiny seeds are powerhouses of excellent nutrients that boosts metabolism and melt fat. They also help to purify and detoxify the body. Soak fennel seeds overnight in water or steep in hot water to make herbal weight loss drink.

Chapter 10: Healthy Veggies and Fruits

Vegetables and fruits are known to be sources of some minerals and vitamins (most especially, Vitamins K and C) that human bodies need to function properly. Examples of minerals that are found in vegetables and fruits include folic acid, potassium, iron and magnesium.

We have been quite pragmatic in choosing those vegetables and fruits that are capable of replenishing the shortage of minerals and vitamins in your body and give you nothing but sound health. Relax but be excited about this list of health-improving veggies and fruits you can lay your hand on at any supermarket near you. The first eight listings are healthy fruits, while the last twelve listings are healthy veggies:

1. **Grapes**

    Grapes contain high quantity of antioxidants and they are useful for reducing cholesterol. You can get them for cheap prices and they are available all year round! It doesn't matter if they are green or purple ones. You can have them alongside salad and other fruits.

2. **Apples**

Do you know why people say eating an apple a day will keep doctors away? This superfood is rich in Vitamin C and antioxidants that can actively fight cancer for you! The red apples seem to be more popular than the green ones, but there is no research finding to prove that red apples are indeed more nutritious than the green ones.

3. **Bananas**

Bananas are low-calorie "snacks", and they are rich in fiber and potassium. Fibers are essential facilitators of metabolism in human bodies. And bananas also contain some amount of water which, when eaten, becomes part of the water in human body. Potassium is an element that normally helps lower the risks of blood pressure, stroke and heart disease. In other words, if you consume banana on a regular basis, you are preparing your body to be ready against diseases like cardiac arrest and stroke.

4. **Kiwi**

Kiwis are indeed an example of berries and they contain fiber and Vitamin C. Vitamin C is generally helpful in maintaining the cell growth and forms a useful protein in skin, ligament, blood vessels and tendons. The fiber part of kiwi fruits is essential for speeding up the metabolism in human body. You can have your kiwi before or after each meal, depending on your preferences.

5. **Cantaloupe**

Cantaloupe is very rich in Vitamin C and they are cheap to obtain. You can be rest assured that the antioxidants a cantaloupe contains can help you maintain a healthy body by slowing your aging process as well as protecting you against any heart disease. If you like, you can mix your cantaloupe with other fruits and vegetables in a bowl of salad.

6. **Watermelons**

Watermelons are another example of superfoods, and they contain in large quantities Vitamin C and antioxidants. Most of the antioxidants can help you fight cancer in order to maintain a healthy body. Watermelons, in some localities, are not seasonal and can be purchased year-round. Make sure your watermelons are not spoilt; it should be fresh red.

7. **Pears**

    Pears are very rich in fiber as well as in Vitamins C. They are reportedly useful in fighting stroke, and eating pears everyday positions your body for better health and longevity. The fiber content of pears affords you the opportunity to speed up your metabolic activities. Pears can be a part of salad or be eaten raw.

8. **Oranges**

    Oranges have been known for ages as the primary source of Vitamin C that our bodies need. However, it also contains in reasonable amount folate, potassium and fiber. The antioxidants in oranges are very helpful in keeping your skin in good shape. As you may have discovered in our fruit listing, we provided fruits that are capable of bringing natural growth to your body cells and help you combat several diseases such as cardiac arrest, overweight, diabetes and poor vision.

    You may decide to have one or two fruits per day, spread over three square meals. Do not overeat these fruits in the hope of filling up your body with a lot of nutrients. Just maintain a balanced-diet approach until you can have all of them within a week or more, depending on their availability and your appetite for fruits. The vegetable listings start from here; we are sure you are familiar with all of them. We refrain from including obscure vegetables in our listing, which readers might have a hard time finding. So, delve right into the list and enjoy yourself reading it!

9. **Garlic**

    Garlic has enviable medicinal benefits, some of which include but are not restricted to the possession of antioxidants, which help our bodies fight heart diseases and Alzheimer's. Garlic is particularly considered as a memory-boosting veggie! So, apart from its horrid smell, garlic also supplies our bodies with useful nutrients.

10. **Canned Pumpkin**

Pumpkins have been known for ages as a real source of antioxidants to human body, and they contain fibers, too, which are very useful in day-to-day metabolic activities. Make sure your canned pumpkin does not contain sodium, which some food companies use as a preservative. Sodium is dangerous to human health.

11. Canned Tomatoes (Diced)

You will get a good amount of antioxidant lycopene when you consume canned tomatoes. If you are thinking of making fast soup or stew, go for canned tomatoes, but make sure no sodium has been added into the tomatoes as a preservative. Fresh tomatoes are also good; the nutrients are expected to still be in their natural states. You can use canned tomatoes to cook soups, prepare salad and serve as an appetizer!

12. Onions

You can use onions in a number of ways: as a condiment in vegan dish or soup. Apart from the sharp sensation it invokes on your tongue, onions are also good sources of antioxidants that prevents heart diseases from affecting you. Use your onions as a part of salad or you even choose to chew it. Do not spit out the whorls of the onions, chew everything and swallow it. It is good for your health!

13. Sweet Potatoes

In addition to its fiber content, sweet potatoes are delicious and very nutritious. They provide Vitamin A to the body and contain beta-carotene, which may hinder the growth of cancerous cells on our skin and protect it from excessive sunlight (tanning). You can decide to make some mashed potatoes or even cooked them as a meal. You may have to combine other vegetables described in this e-book so as to have a great meal.

14. Winter Squash (Acorn, butternut, etc.)

If you are looking for a veggie that can supply your body with freshness, fiber, vitamins and potassium at the same time, go for the winter squash. The primary function of potassium is to help you stay healthy and active by lowering your blood pressure. Imagine how agile you can be when you are not bogged down by a life-threatening high blood pressure!

15. Kale

If you are looking for a veggie that will supply your body with all the necessary fiber, Vitamins C, A and K, and minerals like calcium, potassium and iron, go for Kale. This veggie is like the superstar of all the nutrient-rich ingredients. Eating kale will help your vision, the growth of your body cells and it will speed up your metabolic processes.

16. Broccoli

People have been advised from time to time to eat broccoli to fight cancerous cells in their body. Broccoli is also rich in folate and Vitamin C. When you eat broccoli on a regular basis you are protecting your body against a destructive cancer. You can cook your broccoli as a fresh vegetable or you can include it inside a bowl of salad. No matter your choice, it is important to remember that the bottom line is that you are getting as much nutrient as your body required.

17. Beets

Beets are generally rich in fiber, folate and many vitamins. When you consume beets, you are getting betalains into your body, which is capable of preventing cancer and other body-destroying diseases. Beet can supply magnesium, calcium and iron to your body. Calcium and iron are two elements that are responsible for strengthening some parts of human body, like bones, tendons and muscles.

18. Spinach

Get Vitamins K and A into your body by eating spinach regularly. This green veggie is also a reservoir of minerals like calcium. Vitamins are good for smooth running of the systems in human bodies. Vitamin A, in particular, is good for maintaining good vision. Spinach has always been included in most salad.

19. Carrots

This orange veggie is famous for its nutritious components, which include Vitamin A. This vitamin is particularly useful for enjoying a good vision and maintaining smooth skin. Carrots have zero saturated fat and zero cholesterol. It is a typical weight-loss ingredient and it has a considerable amount of fiber.

20. Edamame

Get it frozen, and you can supply your body with fiber and protein that will help it grow naturally. Edamame is a good source of plant protein! It is a low-calorie vegetable; it also contains Vitamin B complex and calcium. If you want to improve your health, try to eat it at least once a week.

Once again, the good news is that all the healthy fruits and veggies outlined above are cheap to obtain and they are available in all supermarkets all over the world. Get a mix of the fruits and veggies sometimes to increase the amount of minerals and vitamins available to your body at a particular point in time. We do not encourage abusing foods or fruits: eat as much as you feel is good for your body. It is a wrong notion to think that the larger the quantity of food eaten, the bigger the amount of nutrients that would be assimilated into one's body systems.

Food consumption and utilization doesn't work like that; it isn't mathematics that follows a definitive equation formula. Several factors contribute to food utilization in human body: for example, your body systems, your state of health and your willingness to exercise to encourage faster metabolism.

Chapter 11: Healthy Proteins

Proteins are integral part of human body, and they are present in our tissues and organs. Proteins are made up of hundreds or thousands of smaller units called amino acids. Amino acids are found in human hair, nails, tendons and other parts. To strengthen our body systems, we definitely need proteins all the time. Proteins function in different ways in our body: as an antibody for fighting foreign substances that want to attack our health; as an enzyme that facilitates the metabolic processes in our body systems; as a transport/storage facility that helps store up energy for our metabolic activities.

Proteins are obtained from two primary sources: from animals and plants. The healthy proteins included in this e-book are cheap and can be purchased from nearby supermarket. Of course, people don't normally sit down and choose if they were going to buy animal or plant protein. But it is advisable to just mix them up sometimes. Highlighted below are fourteen healthy proteins you can rely on to transform your health. If you are quite serious about maintaining good health in order to live long, you will surely incorporate these recipes into your daily meals:

1. Black beans

Black beans are a good source of cancer-killing antioxidants, fiber, and some minerals like calcium, potassium and folic acid. The dry beans are cheaper and they also have their minerals intact. When you boil your black beans, you are inadvertently preserving the antioxidants from being destroyed.

2. **Eggs**

Eggs are known as quick suppliers of proteins to human bodies. In other words, when your doctor informed you that your body lacks proteins, go get an egg right away and you will be OK. Eggs seem to possess the same nutrients irrespective of their sources, whether from a fowl or a duck.

3. **Almonds**

Almonds contain fiber and monounsaturated fat, the kind of fat that is non-cholesterol in nature. You will probably be advised to eat almonds if you want to fight diabetes and weight-gain. As super-nuts, almonds contribute immensely to the rate of metabolic activity.

4. **Peanuts**

Peanuts may be seen as a fatty food but, if eaten moderately, could supply healthy fat to the body. The legumes are good for fighting heart diseases. As a source of plant protein, it is rich in fiber and antioxidants. Do not be tempted to eat plenty of it; it may surprisingly increase the fat in your body.

5. **Garbanzo beans**

You can have your Garbanzo beans in a powdery form or as a roast. It contains fiber and it is therefore helpful in speeding up metabolism. It also contains some useful vitamins and minerals such as magnesium and calcium. And it has zero cholesterol but it is rich in dietary fiber.

6. **Lentils**

Lentils are used in various meals, as either an ingredient in soup or salad. It is very rich in antioxidants and provides more protein to human body than beef. It tastes good, a quality that makes it popular with vegetarians. Lentils are a low-calorie vegetable and it contains nutrients like calcium, iron and magnesium. The iron and calcium are very useful for strengthening the bones and other structures in human body. Its antioxidant nature helps prevent deadly heart diseases.

7. **Oats**

You may have heard that a bowl of oatmeal is a goldmine of health-improving nutrients. You can get fiber, antioxidants and lower-cholesterol fat. Can you imagine how much nutrient you will be able to give your body if you eat oatmeal as your regular breakfast? It also contains minerals like calcium, magnesium, sodium and potassium. Oats also possess some vitamins such as Vitamin B12, B6, D, K, C and A. Vitamin A is good for maintaining a perfect vision while Vitamin C (ascorbic acid) is good for preventing tanning or undue exposure to sunlight.

8. **Pinto beans**

You can have your pinto beans for breakfast, lunch and dinner. Pinto beans are very rich in fiber and proteins. The fibers are mainly useful for speeding up metabolic processes. Pinto beans have zero calories and it contains elements like iron, Magnesium, and calcium. The beans also possess some good vitamins such as vitamin B complex, C, D and K, all of which are very helpful in maintaining good health. Do not be afraid to eat these beans in any of your meals, whether during breakfast or other times.

9. **Tofu**

Tofu is a soymeal, rich in huge amount of protein but low in fat. Its low-cholesterol characteristic makes it a darling among vegetarians. When consumed moderately, its fiber and antioxidants can reduce cholesterol and the danger of breast cancer.

10. **Pumpkin seeds**

If you lack iron, protein and other vitamins in your body, pumpkin seeds can help you replenish them. You can decide to ground it into a powder form or eat it like roasted seeds.

11. **Chicken breasts**

A good chicken breast contains lean protein, and you don't have to ever worry about putting on weight when you consumed it. It is important to state that quantity matters: eat a moderate size of the chicken breast and you will just be fine.

12. Canned salmon

Eat canned salmon to supply your body with the required protein. Canned salmon comes with different flavors, but make sure you select the one with less chemical (food additives) in it.

13. Canned tuna

The good things about canned tuna is that it is cheap and can provide your body with Omega-3's, which are believed to make people intelligent.

14. Whey protein

Whey protein can be a good supply of protein to human body when consumed with other foods. For example, you can add it to your bowl of oatmeal or custard.

All the healthy proteins described above are very helpful in speeding up metabolism in humans, and they can be a great anti-aging and anti-cancer agent. Do not be afraid to seek medical assistance from your physician if you do not know which food ingredients will be good for your body or not.

Chapter 12: Healthy Drinks

There are countless drinks around us that are quite unhealthy: they fill up our bodies with excess sugar, fat and cholesterol. In order to remain healthy, it is your singular responsibility to make sure that you only consume drinks that are beneficial to your health, the ones that produce no negative side-effects in your body. A drink may be regarded as healthy if:

- It doesn't produce too much sugar, fat, cholesterol
- It doesn't contain dangerous additives
- If it is non-alcoholic in nature
- If it facilitates the process of metabolism
- If it is instrumental to weight-loss and mental soberness

The healthy drinks described in this e-book meet all the criteria listed above, and they also contain additional properties that could be regarded to as health-boosting. Listed below are three main drinks you can drink on a daily basis:

- **Coffee**

    Even though it is true that coffee contains caffeine, which is the major reason most people avoid drinking it, but technically, coffee is also a good source of antioxidants which prevent the heart from experiencing cardiac problems. Think of coffee as a fuel for your body when you work out. Home-brewed coffee is more reliable than the one bought from the vending machine or coffee shop. You may not be able to ascertain which ingredients were used in brewing the coffee bought from the coffee shop. Desist from consuming a lot of coffee per day: having a large quantity of caffeine in your blood stream is absolutely bad for your health.

- **Tea**

    Tea is reputable for supplying human body with the much-needed antioxidants. Researchers believe that the greener a tea, the more the amount of antioxidants it could release into human body. As long as you didn't put a lot of sugar into your tea, you can enjoy its natural flavor and smell. Drinking green tea, for example, has been noted to improve drinker's immune system and help in maintaining weight. This weight-loss property of green tea is why many people are turning to it as a vital drink to rejuvenate their body system.

- **Water**

    We have all seen water as a free substance, which is true to a certain extent. Water is very important for our consumption because human body consists of seventy percent (70%) of water. Water functions as a hydrating liquid that keeps the balance of the metabolites inside the blood stream. Water also helps in flushing out toxic substances from our bodies. If you want to lose weight, drinking some cups of water everyday can position you for a smooth weight-loss process.

Whatever you chose to drink, always remember that you must pay serious attention to the quantity as well as the regularity of consumption. Too much of everything is bad: make sure you consume only the quantity you needed.

Chapter 13: Healthy Whole Grains

Whole grains are notable examples of carbohydrates, and they contain high percentage of dietary fibers per gram. They are also rich in Vitamin B complex (thiamin, riboflavin, niacin and folate). They are noticeable reservoir of life-enriching minerals such as iron, magnesium and selenium.

The primary benefits of whole grains include reducing the chance of contracting a heart disease and facilitating metabolic activities. If your meal lack whole grains like rice, corns and the others, you better run to the nearest supermarket and grab them. They are very useful for maintaining good health, as you will discover shortly. In this book, we list three essential whole-grain foods for your consumption:

- **Whole-grain pasta**

    This white, whole-grain pasta is full of some essential substances like proteins, antioxidants and fiber. When you eat, you aren't only building the cells in your body in a healthy way, but also keeping yourself from having a heart disease.

- **Brown rice**

    Brown rice is usually preferred to the white one because it contains a sizeable amount of fiber that is necessary for reducing the risk of diabetes. Most restaurants go for brown rice because of this unique characteristic.

- **Popcorn**

    Popcorns are a good source of dietary fiber, and it is always advisable that you to go for the low-calorie ones. Do not mess up your popcorn with too much sugar and other unhealthy additives that some people often add to it.

Chapter 14: Healthy Dairy

While it is a good idea to consume some diary from time to time, the right way to do it is by going for low-fat ones. From milk to yoghurt to cheese, dairy products have been noticed as the main sources of vitamins such as B1, B2, B6, B12, A, E and D and important nutrients like proteins, calcium, folate and magnesium. Like every other type of food that we consume, here are some significant reasons why people should consume dairy products regularly:

- To replenish our body systems with protein and calcium
- To obtain vitamin D, which is responsible for lowering the risk of cancer
- Calcium from dairy foods are useful for increasing bone density
- Consuming low-fat dairy products prevents high blood pressure from occurring

- Metabolic syndrome, which causes enlarged waists in people, can only affect people who do not eat dairy products
- Dairy products are useful for weight-loss plans

Highlighted below are three important dairy products you can find in any supermarket near you:

- **Yoghurt**

    Low-calorie yoghurt is the best choice if you want to maximize the amount of protein and calcium you can derive from it. This type of yoghurt is even helpful in losing weight. Make it your habit to eat it once a day, most especially as part of your breakfast menu.

- **Low-fat milk**

    Drink low-fat milk whenever you need to add more calcium and protein to your body system. You can keep your teeth and bone strong by using the calcium supplied by this milk.

- **Cottage cheese**

    Cottage cheese is rich in proteins and calcium. It is advisable you go for the low-fat or fat-free one. Cheese often tastes good and you can apply it to different types of meals you have in a day.

Chapter 15: Recipe Meals

1. Herbal Arugula Soup

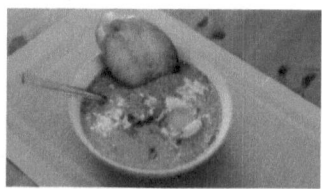

This soup is loaded with antioxidants and is simply as good hot as it is cold. And 1 cup of this soup is just 88 calories.

Ingredients

- 2 (5 oz.) containers of baby arugula
- 1 tbsp. of olive oil

- 1 medium onion, chopped
- 1 tsp of cornstarch
- 2 cloves of garlic, chopped
- 6 cups of chicken broth, low-sodium
- ½ cup of evaporated milk, low-fat
- ¼ cup of mixed herbs (like mint, parsley, chives, and tarragon), chopped
- 4 tbsp. of Greek yogurt, plain
- 2 tbsp. of sliced chives

Method

1. In a saucepan, heat olive oil on medium-low heat. Add garlic and onion and cook till translucent for about 5 minutes. Stir in cornstarch, evaporated milk and chicken broth; bring it to simmer.

2. Add mixed herbs and arugula and stir till wilted; cover and set aside 5 minutes. Use an immersion blender to blend until smooth. Divide among 6 bowls; garnish each with 2 tsp plain Greek yogurt and 1 tsp sliced chives.

Good to know

Arugula is amazingly low in calories, saturated fat, fat, and cholesterol. It is, however, loaded with fibre, vitamins A, C and K, and other essential nutrients, including potassium.

2. Broccoli Omelet with Toast

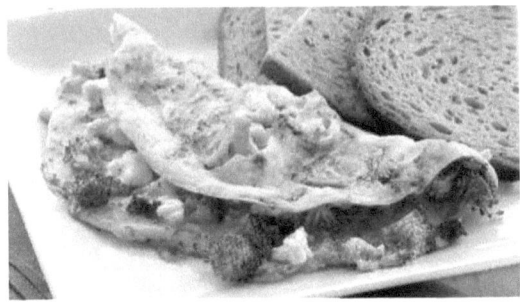

Broccoli is a super food and is remarkably low in calories. It is loaded with fiber, essential minerals and vitamins, and powerful antioxidants.

Ingredients

- 1 cup of broccoli, chopped
- Cooking spray
- 2 large eggs, beaten
- ¼ tsp of dry dill
- 2 tbsp. of feta cheese, crumbled
- 2 slices of rye bread, toasted

Method

1. Coat a non-stick pan with some cooking spray on medium heat. Add broccoli and cook for about 3 minutes.

2. Whisk egg, dill, and feta in a bowl. Add this egg mixture to the pan. Cook for about 3-4 minutes; turn the omelette; cook for 2 minutes or till cooked through. Serve the omelette with toast.

Good to know

We can use either frozen or fresh broccoli. Both work simply fine. The feta cheese gives a punch of flavor. The chemical present in broccoli gives it a slightly bitter flavor.

3. Lettuce and Chicken Salad

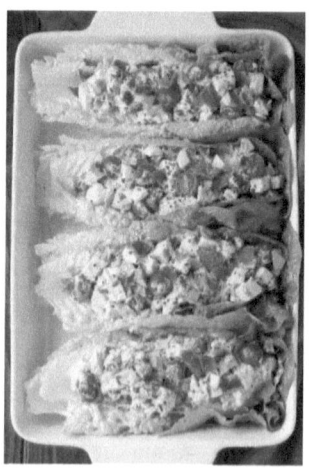

We can eat lots of lettuce (of any variety) without gaining any extra ounce. Romaine lettuce is also a great source of vitamin B, manganese, and folic acid.

Ingredients

- 3 cups of romaine lettuce, chopped
- 1 cup of potatoes, cubed (½-inch cubes)
- 1/8 tsp of salt
- 1/8 tsp of pepper
- Cooking spray
- 2 tbsp. of water
- 2 tbsp. of lime juice
- 1 tsp of honey
- 1 tsp of fresh ginger, peeled and grated
- 2 tbsp. of peanuts, chopped
- 1 tsp of dark sesame-oil
- 2 oz. of skinless chicken, grilled or baked and chopped
- 1 tbsp. of fresh mint, chopped
- 1 tbsp. of fresh cilantro, chopped

Method

1. Spray the potato with little bit of cooking spray. Place it in microwave-safe dish and sprinkle with salt and pepper. Add 2 tbsp. of water and cover; microwave it on HIGH for 5 minutes or till tender.

2. Mix oil, honey, lime juice, and ginger in a bowl and stir well. Combine lettuce, potato, chicken, mint, peanuts, and cilantro in a mixing bowl. Add the honey dressing and gently toss to coat.

Good to know

If we are short in time, we can use precooked chicken strips or rotisserie chicken and/or bottled sesame-ginger dressing for this recipe.

4. Grapefruit Avocado and Salmon Salad

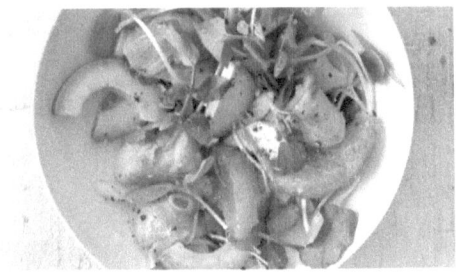

Grapefruit helps us in fast weight loss by curbing our hunger and it also lowers our cholesterol.

Ingredients

- 3 (5 oz.) wild salmon-fillets (skin on)
- 1 large grapefruit
- 2 large bunches (10 cups) of arugula, stems removed
- 2 tbsp. of lemon juice
- 1 ripe avocado, pitted, sliced
- 2 tbsp. of olive oil
- ½ tsp of black pepper, freshly grounded, divided
- ½ tsp of kosher salt, divided
- Cooking spray
- ¼ cup of walnuts, toasted roughly chopped

Method

1. Peel and slice the grapefruit; reserve the juice in one bowl. Toss grapefruit slices and juice with avocado and arugula; divide the salad into serving plates. In a bowl, combine together oil, lemon juice, and ¼ tsp of each of salt and pepper.

2. Sprinkle the remaining salt and pepper on both sides of fillet. Heat a non-stick skillet on medium-high heat and Coat it with cooking spray. Add fillet (with skin-side down) to the skillet; cook till skin becomes golden for about 4 minutes.

3. Gently turn the fish; cook for about 3 more minutes. Break each fish into 4 pieces; top the salads each with 3 fish pieces. Drizzle the salads with the reserved dressing and sprinkle with some walnuts.

Good to know

Salmon and walnuts contain omega-3 fatty acids and avocado is rich in monounsaturated fats which are good for heart.

5. Mushrooms with Vegetable Stuffing

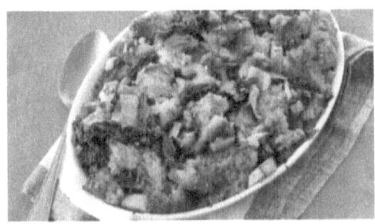

Mushrooms are incredibly low-cal and contain immune-boosting antioxidants, together with B vitamins, potassium, and fibre.

Ingredients

- 4 large Portobello-mushroom caps
- 2 tsp of olive oil
- ¼ tsp of coarse salt
- 1½ tbsp. of balsamic vinegar
- ½ tsp of black pepper, freshly grounded, divided
- 1/3 cup of Kalamata olives, chopped
- 1½ cups of tomato, chopped
- 1 cup of whole-grain breadcrumbs, fresh
- ¼ cup of fresh chives, chopped
- ½ cup (4 oz.) of fontina cheese, shredded

Method

1. Preheat the oven at 400°. Place the mushroom caps, with gill side up, on baking sheet; drizzle with vinegar and oil, and season them with salt to taste and ¼ tsp of pepper. Bake them in oven till mushrooms become tender, for about 10 minutes.

2. In the meanwhile, mix olives, tomato, breadcrumbs, chives, and cheese in a bowl. Season it with the remaining ¼ tsp of pepper. Evenly divide the vegetable mixture (about ½ cup per cap) into mushroom caps. Bake them for 10-12 minutes or till mushrooms become tender and lightly browned. Serve them hot.

Good to know

Mushrooms are loaded also with proteins, folate, and potassium.

6. Crispy and Cheesy Zucchini Rings

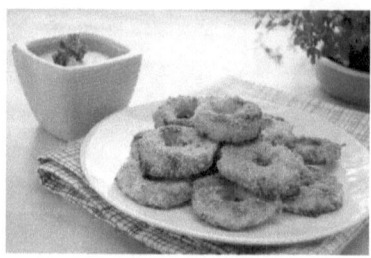

Zucchini is the ultimate high-volume food, i.e., we can fill up on extremely few calories. It is packed with lots of vitamin A.

Ingredients

- 2 zucchinis
- ¼ tsp of salt
- 2 oz. (about 24) of sun-dried tomatoes, packed in oil
- 3 oz. of goat cheese
- ¼ tsp of black pepper, freshly grounded
- 2 tbsp. of fresh chives, chopped
- 2 tbsp. of extra-virgin olive-oil

Method

1. Cut zucchini into slices of ¼-inch thickness. Place them on a plate; season them with salt and pepper. Place 1 tomato on every slice, then top every tomato with a little bit of goat cheese. Sprinkle with chives over the tops, drizzle with olive oil and serve.

Good to know

Zucchini is very simple to prepare raw or to cook with!

7. Grapefruit and Kale Salad

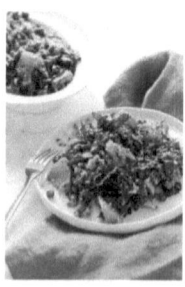

The star ingredient in this salad is grapefruit. It is one of the top super-foods for weight-loss.

Ingredients

- 2 pink grapefruits
- ½ red onion, sliced thinly, divided
- ½ cup of fat-free yogurt, plain
- 2 tbsp. of extra-virgin olive-oil
- ¼ cup of lemon juice, fresh
- ½ tsp of kosher salt
- ¼ tsp of black pepper
- 1 oz. (1/3 cup) of hazelnuts, toasted and chopped
- 8 oz. of lacinato kale, sliced very thinly

Method

1. Peel and slice the grapefruit; reserve 3 tbsp. of juice in a bowl. Chop 2 onion rings. Add them to grapefruit juice, along with oil, yogurt, lemon juice, salt, and pepper. Whisk till well mixed. Toss in chopped kale. Top with grapefruit, hazelnuts, and remaining onion.

Good to know

There are a lot of super-foods present in this delicious salad. Kale consists of vitamins A, C, and K, and grapefruit helps in fast weight-loss by cutting our hunger and it also lowers cholesterol.

8. Chocolate Chip Pumpkin Bread

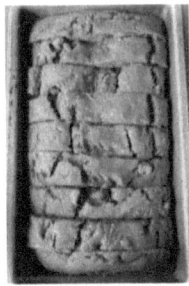

Pumpkin is a low-calorie squash and is loaded with potassium and rich in beta-carotene (a powerful antioxidant), and its natural sweetness provides flavor to baked items without any extra guilt.

Ingredients

- 2 cups of sugar
- 2 cups of canned pumpkin
- ½ cup of vanilla pudding, (fat-free)
- 4 large egg-whites
- ½ cup of canola oil
- 3 cups of all-purpose flour
- 2 tsp of cinnamon, ground
- 1 tsp of baking soda
- 1¼ tsp of salt
- 1 cup of semi-sweet chocolate chips
- Cooking spray

Method

1. Preheat the oven at 350°. Combine sugar, pumpkin, canola oil, vanilla pudding and egg-whites in a bowl, whisking well. Mix flour, salt, baking soda and cinnamon in another bowl, whisking well. Add this flour mixture to the pumpkin mixture and stir just till moist. Stir in the chocolate chips.

2. Spoon the batter into loaf pan greased with the cooking spray. Bake in oven at 350° for about 1 hour 15 minutes or till a tooth-pick inserted in center comes out cleanly. Allow the bread to cool in pan for 10 minutes on the wire rack; remove it from pan. Cool it completely on the wire rack.

Good to know

Substituting egg whites in place of whole eggs keeps this bread cholesterol-free plus cuts saturated fat by half, while the pumpkin which is rich in fibre provides us with the entire day's vitamin A requirement just with 1 slice. Opt for dark-chocolate chips (prepared without milk) with a minimum of 60% cocoa for antioxidant boost.

9. Radish and Cucumber Fry with Noodles

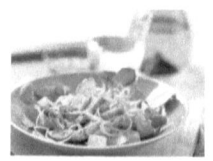

This is a low-cholesterol and low-saturated fat recipe. So, it can be used for weight loss.

Ingredients

- 7 oz. of dry rice noodles
- 1 tbsp. of canola oil
- 1 large cucumber, thinly sliced
- ¾ tsp of salt, divided
- 1 cup of radishes, thinly sliced
- ¼ cup of hoisin sauce
- 2 tbsp. of soy sauce, low-sodium
- 7 cups (about 3 bunches) of watercress, trimmed
- ¼ tsp of cayenne pepper, ground
- 1 tsp of sesame oil
- 1 tsp of sesame seeds, toasted
- 1 cup (6 oz.) of tofu, cut into cubes of ½-inch

Method

1. Cook noodles as per package directions and drain. In the meanwhile, heat canola-oil in a non-stick skillet on medium-high heat. Add cucumber and radish; sauté for 1 minute, or till tender. Stir in ½ tsp of salt, hoisin sauce, soy sauce, cayenne and noodles and sauté for 1 minute.

2. Mix watercress and noodle mixture. Sprinkle the tofu with remaining ¼ tsp of salt. Heat the sesame-oil in a skillet on medium-high heat. Add tofu; sauté for 2 minutes. Place tofu on noodle mixture. Sprinkle it with sesame seeds.

Good to know

Radishes are rich in nutrients (both root and greens). Radish greens are rich in vitamin C, calcium and potassium.

10. Spicy Green Tea

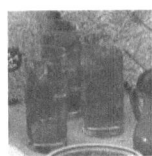

Caffeine and catechin (an antioxidant) present in green tea increase fat-burning, so green tea helps us in shedding pounds.

Ingredients

- ¾ cup of green tea, strong and chilled
- 1/8 tsp of cayenne pepper
- 2 tsp of agave nectar
- 1 small pear (skin on), cut
- 2-3 tbsp. of lemon juice
- 2 tbsp. of fat-free yogurt, plain
- 6-8 ice cubes

Method

1. Put all the ingredients in the blender. Blend till smooth and serve chilled.

Good to know

All teas are rich in polyphenol, an antioxidant which protects cells from DNA damage and they also lower bad cholesterol, boost brain power, and keep us thin.

11. Celery Root and Apple Salad

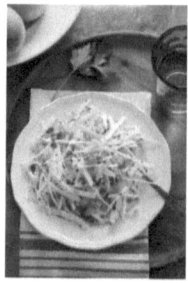

This fresh salad is easy to prepare and it has not more than 100 calories so we can splurge over its tasty flavors.

Ingredients

- ¼ cup of low-fat buttermilk
- 1 oz. of blue cheese, crumbled
- ½ tsp of Worcestershire sauce

- 3 dashes of hot pepper-sauce (like Tabasco)
- 3 tbsp. of chives, chopped (plus extra for garnishing)
- ¼ tsp of black pepper, freshly grounded
- 3 tbsp. of lemon juice, fresh
- ½ lb. of celery root, peeled, cut into strips (about 1 cup)
- 2 Granny-Smith apples

Method

1. Whisk buttermilk, cheese, chives, Worcestershire sauce, pepper sauce and black pepper together. Toss the celery root strips with this buttermilk dressing; allow it to stand for 15 minutes.

2. In the meanwhile, cut the apples into slices crosswise and core with a knife. Toss apple slices with lemon juice to prevent browning. Beginning with the apple slices, stack apple alternately with celery mixture on serving plate. Garnish with extra chives, and serve.

Good to know

Celery is packed with fibre and an extremely high-volume food (i.e., can be eaten a lot for a small number of calories).

12. Berry Smoothie

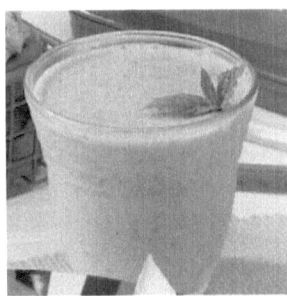

Most of on-the-go smoothies are often filled with sugar and so a lot of calories. But this version saves around 140 calories; in addition, it is packed with antioxidants.

Ingredients

- 1 cup of berries (strawberries, raspberries, or blueberries)
- ¼ cup of pomegranate juice
- ½ banana

- 1 cup of ice cubes
- ¼ cup of water

Method

1. Combine all the ingredients in the blender and blend till smooth.

Good to know

Blueberries, strawberries, raspberries –all are loaded with anti-inflammatories, which lessen the risk of cancer and heart disease. These are antioxidant powerhouses and immunity boosters.

13. Classic Carrot-Ginger Soup

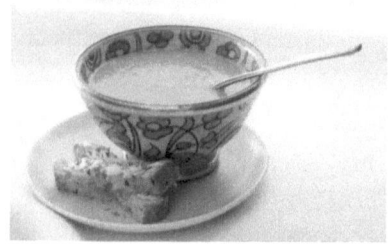

This is a low-carbohydrate, low-cholesterol and low-fat soup. The carrots present in this soup provide tons of beta-carotene nutrients.

Ingredients

- 8 (1 lb.) carrots, sliced,
- 1 tbsp. of fresh ginger, chopped
- ¼ tsp of red pepper, crushed (plus extra for garnishing)
- ½ tsp of kosher salt
- 1 clove of garlic, smashed
- 4 cups of water
- 2 tsp of lemon juice, fresh

Method

1. In a pot, simmer carrots, ginger, garlic, pepper, salt and water, covered, till carrots become tender for 20 to 25 minutes. In a blender (in batches), blend them till smooth; add 2 tsp of lemon juice. Pour the

soup in serving bowls; garnish with carrot leaves and crushed red pepper. Serve it chilled, if desired.

Good to know

Carrot is very low in cholesterol and saturated fat. It is a great source of niacin, thiamine, vitamin B6, dietary fibre, vitamins A C and K and potassium.

14. Oats and Dark Chocolate Clusters

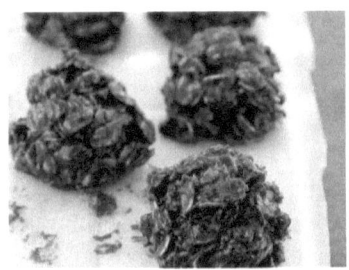

Oats are loaded with fibre, so one serving helps us feel filled throughout day. Just ½ cup of oats packs 4.6 g of resistant-starch that burns fat.

Ingredients

- 2 tbsp. of peanut butter
- 2 tbsp. of 1% low-fat milk
- ¾ cup of old-fashioned rolled oats
- ¼ cup of semi-sweet chocolate chips

Method

1. Heat milk, peanut butter, and chocolate-chips in a pan on low heat for about 3 minutes or till chips melt. Add oats and remove from the heat. With a scoop, drop 8 balls of the oats mixture on a baking sheet lined with wax paper. Allow them to set in refrigerator for about 10 minutes and then serve!

Good to know

Peanut butter and chocolate are both rich in MUFAs. As an additional benefit, the oats provide us with resistant starch.

15. Avocado Tomato and Lettuce Sandwich

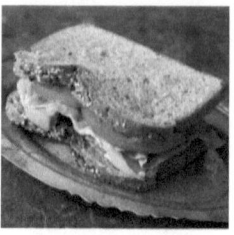

This sandwich is rich in nutrients. Avocado is fattening, but it provides heart-healthy mono-unsaturated fat. Avocado is also rich in fiber. It can be used as healthy cooking and baking substitute for shortening and butter.

Ingredients

- 2 tbsp. of fat-free mayonnaise
- 8 (1 oz.) slices of whole-grain bread with flax seed, toasted
- 1 ripe tomato, sliced thinly
- 1 peeled avocado, sliced
- 4 large leaves of romaine lettuce (or Boston)
- 12 extremely thin slices of cucumber
- 4 (.77 oz.) slices of low-fat, low-sodium Swiss cheese (like Alpine Lace)

Method

1. Spread the mayonnaise over 8 slices of bread. Layer each of 4 slices with 1 leaf of lettuce, 1 tomato slice, 1 avocado slice, 3 cucumber slices, and 1 cheese slice; top each with remaining 4 bread slices. Cut the sandwiches diagonally into half.

Good to know

There is no need to be afraid of consuming fat—so long as it is the right fat. Oleic acid, the compound present in avocados' healthy monounsaturated fats (MUFAs), triggers our body to in fact quiet hunger.

16. Pineapple Salsa and Pan-Grilled Salmon

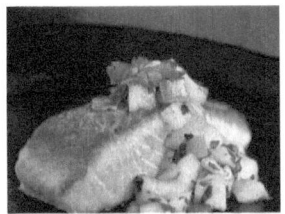

Lean source of protein such as salmon helps us feel filled without adding any fats.

Ingredient

- 1 cup of fresh pineapple, chopped
- 2 tbsp. of red onion, finely chopped
- 1 tbsp. of rice vinegar
- 1/8 tsp of red pepper, ground
- 2 tbsp. of cilantro, chopped
- Cooking spray
- ½ tsp of salt
- 4 (6 oz.) salmon fillets (about ½-inch thick)

Method

1. Combine pineapple, red onion, cilantro, vinegar and red pepper in a mixing bowl and keep aside. Coat a non-stick grill-pan with cooking-spray and heat it on medium-high heat. Sprinkle the fillet with salt. Cook the fillet for 4 minutes on both the sides or till it easily flakes with fork. Top the fillet with pineapple salsa.

Good to know

Salmon is loaded with omega-3 fatty acids. It also adds fibre, which helps digestion.

17. Cheesy Pear

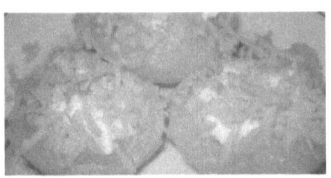

Eating 3 pears per day may result in lower calorie consumption and more weight loss.

Ingredients

- 1 small pear, cut into half and cored
- ¼ tsp of cinnamon, ground
- ¼ cup of ricotta cheese, part-skimmed

Method

1. Preheat toaster oven or broiler. Place the pear on baking sheet and broil for about 10 to 12 minutes till it becomes tender. Combine cinnamon and ricotta cheese in a bowl. Top the pear with the ricotta mixture and serve warm!

Good to know

This snack is rich in both CLA and fibre. The fibre hides in its skin. The cinnamon helps control blood sugar, too.

18. Citrus and Ginger Salad

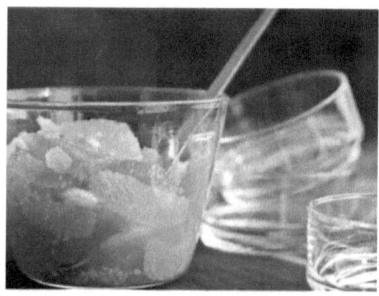

Even if we do not change anything else about our diet, eating ½ grapefruit prior to each meal helps us lose a pound per week!

Ingredients

- 1 pink grapefruit
- Fresh ginger
- 3 oranges
- 1 tbsp. of honey
- Fresh mint, for garnishing

Method

1. Peel and slice the grapefruit and peel and segment 2 oranges. Juice the remaining orange. Grate 2 tsp of ginger, and add it to orange juice and honey in a bowl. Place orange segments in serving bowl; drizzle with honey mixture. Refrigerate it for 1 hour, and serve as it is or serve it over low-fat ice cream. Garnish it with mint, if you like.

Good to know

A compound in the grapefruit lowers insulin (fat-storage hormone), and which in turn leads to weight-loss. It is a great source of protein too, and as it is filled with 90% of water, it fills us up so we eat less.

19. Almond French Toast

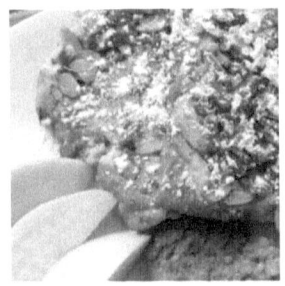

Nuts are rich in healthy fats which help us slim down. Almonds in particular help us shed pounds.

Ingredients

- 1 large egg
- 2 large egg-whites
- 3 tbsp. of sugar
- ¼ tsp of vanilla extract, pure
- 1/8 tsp of salt
- ¼ tsp of almond extract
- 1¼ cups of 1% low-fat milk
- 8 (1-inch) slices of round Italian bread (ciabatta)
- ¼ cup of whole milk
- Cooking spray
- 1 cup of almonds, sliced

Method

1. Heat a griddle on medium-low heat. Whisk 1 egg, 2 egg-whites, salt, sugar, vanilla extract and almond extract together in a bowl. Gradually stir in both the milks. Pour the mixture into one shallow baking pan. Soak the bread in the pan for 3 minutes on both sides.

2. Coat the griddle with cooking-spray. For every slice of bread, place 2 tbsp. of almonds in a layer on hot griddle and press one side of bread into almonds; cook for 4 minutes or till golden brown. Turn the bread; cook for 3–4 minutes or till golden brown. Serve immediately.

Good to know

Adding nuts (almonds in particular) to a low-calorie diet daily may help in more weight loss.

20. Minty Ice Tea

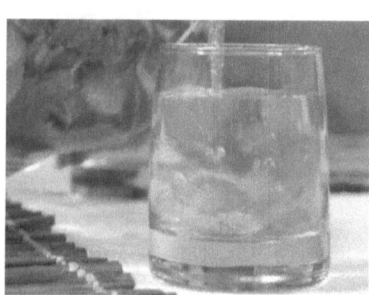

Green tea helps us fill up and shed pounds. In addition, the antioxidants present in green-tea will increase our calorie burn and fat burn.

Ingredients

- 1 cup of mint leaves, fresh
- Ice
- 3-4 green-tea bags
- Honey or agave, (optional)
- Fresh lavender leaves (optional)

Method

1. Put mint leaves in one glass pitcher. Gently crush them with hands. Add tea bags to it; pour hot-water over the top. Cover it and keep in

fridge for about 4-6 hours. Remove the tea bags; serve it over ice. Add agave or honey to sweeten the tea and some fresh lavender leaves.

Good to know

One study revealed that 5 cups of green tea per day helps us lose two times as much weight.

21. Brown Lentil Soup

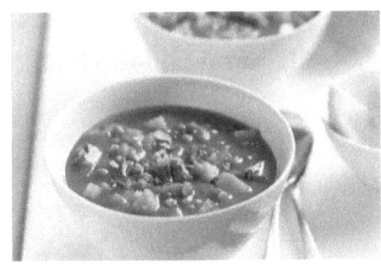

Lentils are a good source of satisfying protein and fibre. ½ cup of serving delivers 3.4 g of the resistant starch, one healthy carb which burns fat.

Ingredients

- 2 tsp of olive oil
- 3 carrots, chopped
- 2 tsp of fresh ginger, peeled and grated
- 1 tsp of garlic, minced
- 1 onion, chopped
- 1½ tsp of curry powder
- ¼ tsp of black pepper, freshly ground
- ¼ tsp of salt
- 4 cups of water
- 2 (14 oz.) cans of fat-free, low-sodium chicken broth,
- 1 cup of brown lentils, washed and drained
- 1 (14.5 oz.) can of diced tomatoes, drained

Method

1. Heat olive-oil in a pan on medium heat. Add onion and carrot and cover; cook for 3 minutes or till softened. Add garlic and ginger and cook for 1 minute. Add curry powder, pepper, and salt and cook for 30 seconds.

2. Add chicken broth, water and lentils; bring it to boil. Reduce the heat; simmer it, covered, for 20 to 25 minutes or till lentils become tender. Add tomatoes and cover; simmer for 5 minutes and serve.

Good to know

Lentils are a great source of protein and fibre. But when they are boiled, many of nutrients go away into water, so using them in a soup form like this, is a better way to retain all those nutrients.

22. Duck-Confit and Blood Orange Salad

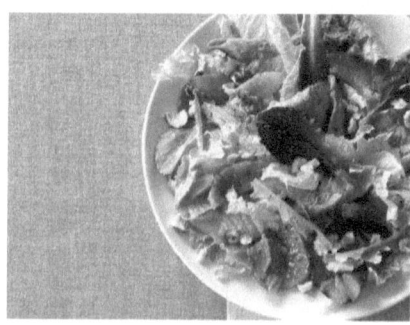

Orange being highest source of fibre is great filling food. Feeling full helps us eat less during the entire day.

Ingredients

- 1 tbsp. of sherry vinegar
- 4 blood oranges, divided (3 segmented and 1 juiced)
- 1 tbsp. of olive oil
- ¼ tsp of salt
- 1 tsp of Dijon mustard
- ¼ tsp of pepper
- 6 cups of mixed winter greens (such as spinach, lettuce, and escarole)
- 1 duck-confit leg (5-6 oz.), shredded, skin, bones and fat discarded (about ¾ cup)
- ¼ cup of skinned hazelnuts, toasted and chopped

Method

1. In a bowl, combine orange juice, vinegar, mustard, and olive-oil and mix well. Add salt and pepper. In another bowl, mix salad greens,

hazelnuts, shredded duck, and orange sections. Drizzle with salad dressing and serve.

Good to know

Similar to all other citrus fruits, blood orange is a good source of fibre and vitamin C. In addition, anthocyanin present in it is a great antioxidant.

23. Pan-Fried Pine Nuts and Brussels Sprouts

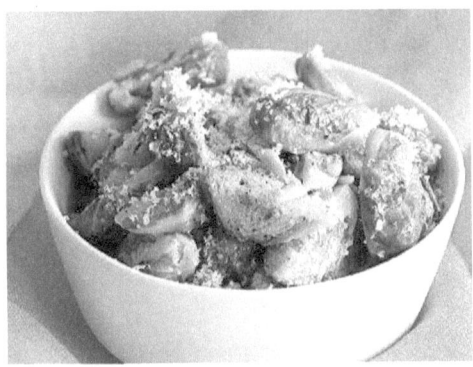

Pine nuts are loaded with some heart-healthy unsaturated fatty acids which suppress hunger hormones and also burn fat. Swapping saturated fatty acids with unsaturated fatty acids helps in weight reduction without reducing intake of calories.

Ingredients

- 1 ½ tbsp. of olive oil
- 1 ½ lb. of Brussels sprouts, thinly sliced
- ½ tsp of black pepper, freshly ground
- 1 tsp of sea salt
- ¼ cup of red-wine vinegar
- 2 tbsp. of pine nuts, toasted
- ¼ cup of Parmesan shavings

Method

1. Heat olive-oil in a non-stick skillet on medium heat; add Brussels-sprouts, pepper, and salt. Cook till sprouts become golden and tender for about 6 minutes, stirring in between.

2. Remove the skillet from heat; add red-wine vinegar and toss well. Transfer sprouts to serving bowl; top them with pine nuts and Parmesan.

Good to know

Brussels sprouts are loaded with nutrients. They pair well with pine nuts and Parmesan. This recipe is full of flavour, but with very low calories.

24. Chocolate-Milk Shake

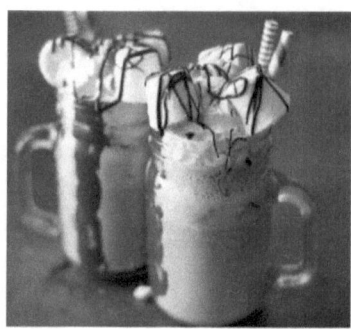

Cocoa powder consists of more antioxidants than the regular chocolate or chocolate-syrup. So, it gives this milk shake a heart-healthy kick.

Ingredients

- 1 cup of low-fat chocolate flavored frozen yogurt
- 1 tbsp. of unsweetened cocoa-powder
- 1 cup of 1% low-fat milk
- 1 tbsp. of agave syrup

Method

1. Place all the ingredients in the blender; blend them till smooth and serve!

Good to know

The fatty acid found in milk, and milk's proteins keeps us feeling satisfied. The calcium also helps in burning fats and calories.

25. Roasted Quinoa with Corn

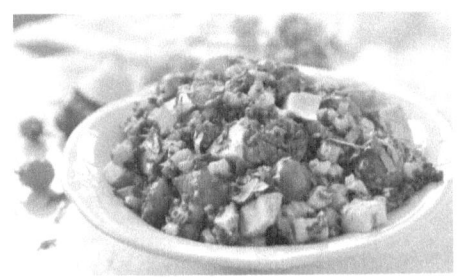

Quinoa is one more diet-friendly whole grain and is loaded with hunger-fighting protein. We'll stay filled longer for fewer calories.

Ingredients

- 1 cup of quinoa, uncooked
- 1 tsp of cumin, ground
- 1 tsp of unsweetened cocoa
- 1 (14 oz.) can of fat-free, low-sodium chicken broth
- ½ tsp of salt
- 1 cup of canned whole-kernel corn, drained (no salt-added)
- ¼ cup of scallions, thinly sliced
- 1/3 cup of jalapeño peppers, chopped
- 2 tbsp. of lime juice

Method

1. Place quinoa in a pan with tight-fitting lid; place pan on high heat. Swirl quinoa to toast evenly. When they crackle and are fragrant, remove the pan from the heat. Add salt, cocoa, and, cumin; then add the broth slowly. Put pan on high heat and bring it to boil.

2. Reduce the heat to a low; cook, covered, for about 15 minutes or till liquid gets absorbed. Add jalapeño peppers and corn and cover; cook for 2 minutes more. Stir in lime juice and scallions and serve warm.

Good to know

This recipe is low in cholesterol and low in saturated fat.

26. Avocado & Egg Toast

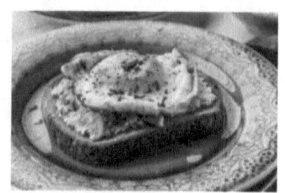

If you thought you didn't have time for a healthy breakfast, this recipe proves you wrong. It comes complete with a good dose of fiber, protein, and healthy unsaturated fats.

Ingredients

- 1 Avocado
- 1 tsp Lemon Juice
- Salt & Pepper to taste
- 2 Whole Eggs (cooked to your liking)
- 2 slices Whole Grain Bread (toasted)
- Black Beans (optional)
- Tomatoes (optional)
- Grated Cheddar Cheese (optional)

Method

1. Toast bread to liking. Mash avocado and lemon juice with a fork. Cook eggs to liking. Spread avocado across toast. Top with eggs. Salt and pepper to taste. Optional: Before putting on eggs, add tomato slices, grated cheddar, and warmed black beans.

Health Facts

This simple and quick breakfast is high in fiber which is great for your health. Eating at least 25-30 grams of fiber daily can help improve digestion and burn more fat. It also helps clear up skin by detoxing and cleansing the body!

27. Breakfast Burrito

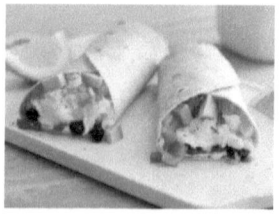

Enjoy your breakfast burritos guilt free by using this perfectly healthy recipe. Make a big batch of them on the weekend and freeze them for a quick and satisfying breakfast throughout the week.

Ingredients

- 3 Eggs
- ¼ cup canned Black Beans (drained)
- 2 Tbsps. Salsa
- 2 Tbsps. Grated Cheddar
- 1 Whole Grain Tortilla

Method

1. Scramble together eggs, cheese, beans, and salsa. Spoon into tortilla. Fold. Enjoy.

Health Facts

This simple recipe is extremely versatile. Add in more veggies or change up the type of beans to keep things interesting and get a varied diet.

Eggs are a great source of protein as well as just about every vitamin and mineral you need.

Whole grain tortillas and black beans provide an energy dose of fiber.

28. Banana Carrot Muffins

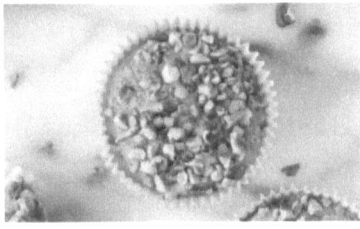

Banana and carrot add a rich yet subtle sweetness to these delicious muffins. They are perfect for an on-the-go breakfast or a mid-day snack.

Ingredients

- 1 ¼ cups Whole Grain Flour
- ½ cup Mashed Banana

- ½ tsp Baking Soda
- ½ tsp Baking Powder
- ½ tsp Nutmeg
- ½ tsp Salt
- 1 cup Rolled Oats
- ½ cup Raisins
- 1 ripe Banana (mashed)
- 4 carrots (grated)
- 1/3 cup Whole Milk
- 1 large Egg
- Olive Oil

Method

1. Preheat oven to 400°F. Grease 12-cup muffin pan with olive oil. In a large bowl, whisk together first 6 ingredients until blended. Stir in raisins and oats. Stir in 3 tablespoons olive oil, milk, egg, banana, and carrot. Stir until blended. Divide batter evenly among 12 muffin cups. Bake 20-25 minutes or until inserted toothpick comes out clean.

Health Facts

This recipe is so scrumptious, you won't even notice it's totally sugar free. Don't be afraid to chow down guilt-free.

Studies have shown that people who eat little sugar (less than 10% of their total calories) can burn up to 365 more calories per day than those who eat more sugar.

These muffins are packed with vitamins and minerals that will keep your bones and muscles strong.

29. Ham & Cheese Quinoa Bites

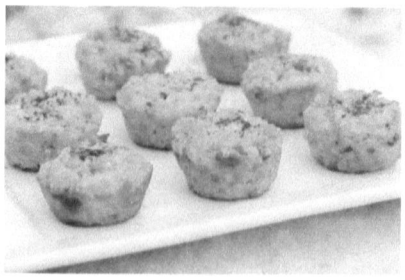

Ham, cheese, and quinoa turn these breakfast nibbles into a powerful protein boost that are perfect for starting the day off right (or giving yourself a quick pick-me-up in the afternoon).

Ingredients

- 2 cups Quinoa (cooked)
- 4 Eggs
- 1 cup Zucchini (grated)
- 1 cup Grated Cheddar
- ½ cup Ham (diced)
- ¼ cup Parsley (chopped)
- 2 Tbsps. Parmesan
- 2 Green Onions (sliced)
- Salt & Pepper to taste

Method

1. Preheat oven to 350°F. Liberally coat muffin tin with oil. Combine all ingredients in a large bowl until well mixed. Divide mixture evenly into muffin cups. Bake 15-20 minutes (or until edges are golden). Let cool 5 minutes.

2. Make ahead and freeze by placing baked quinoa bites on a tray and setting in the freezer until frozen. Then, transfer frozen bites to a freezer bag and store until ready to eat. Reheat in microwave for 20-40 seconds.

Health Facts

With a high dose of protein, these easy to make bites are perfect just before (or just after) a workout.

Zucchini and onions provide plenty of vitamins and minerals along with fiber making these a perfectly balanced meal in miniature. Don't be afraid to experiment with different combinations of veggies and meats.

Use the quinoa base to create nutritious bites that meat your health needs.

30. Cranberry Quinoa Muffins

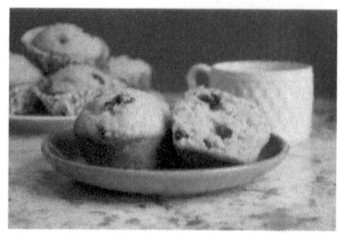

Quinoa takes over the work of flour in these scrumptious and satisfying breakfast muffins.

Ingredients

- 1 cup Quinoa
- 3 Tbsps. Olive Oil
- 2 cups Whole Grain Flour
- ¾ cup Mashed Banana
- 1 ½ tsp Baking Powder
- ½ tsp Salt
- ½ cup Dried Cranberries
- ¾ cup Whole Milk
- 1 large Egg
- 1 tsp Vanilla Extract

Method

1. Submerge quinoa fully in water. Bring to a boil. Reduce heat. Simmer until water is absorbed and quinoa is fluffy. Preheat oven to 350°F. Grease a muffin tin with oil. Dust with flour.

2. In a large bowl, whisk together flour, salt, baking powder, dried cranberries, and 2 cups of the quinoa. Reserve remaining quinoa for later use.

3. In another bowl, whisk together milk, egg, oil, banana, and vanilla. Stir milk mixture into flour mixture until just combined. Divide batter evenly into muffin cups. Bake for 25-30 minutes or until inserted toothpick comes out clean.

Health Facts

Quinoa is a high protein, high fiber grain that can be used in place of flour, rice, and other grains for a healthier meal.

These muffins are not only sugar free but they contain a serious dose of protein, fiber, and healthy unsaturated fats! These are the perfect between meal snacks.

Cranberries are packed with cancer-preventing antioxidants!

31. Pumpkin Oatmeal

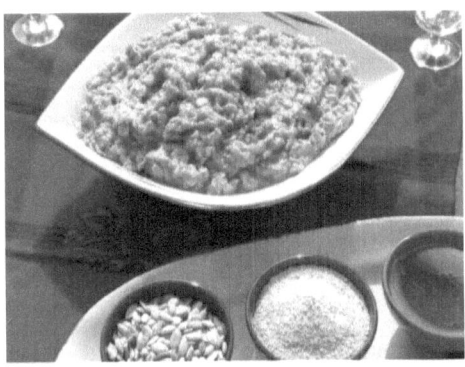

Pumpkin puree and spice adds more nutrition and richer flavor to your heart-healthy oatmeal breakfast.

Ingredients

- 1 ¾ cups Coconut or Almond Milk
- ½ cup Rolled Oats
- ½ cup Pumpkin Puree
- ½ tsp Pumpkin Pie Spice
- Salt to taste
- Almonds & Coconut Flakes (optional)

Method

1. In a pot, boil milk. Stir in the next 4 ingredients. Reduce heat to medium-low. Let simmer until oats are cooked. Sprinkle chopped almonds (or pecans) and unsweetened coconut flakes to serve.

Health Facts

Pumpkin is a great source of vitamin A, E, K, Iron, Magnesium, Potassium, and countless other vitamins and minerals so make this oatmeal recipe part of your morning routine.

Oatmeal is high in protein and fiber. It's also extremely versatile so you can use it in just about anything! Studies have shown that eating oatmeal on a daily basis helps lower blood pressure and reduce your risk of heart attack.

32. Avocado Wraps

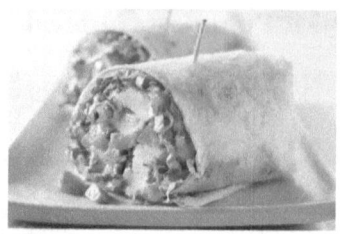

The rich, creamy flavor of avocado is the star of this easy to make lunch wrap.

Ingredients

- 1 cup Chicken (cooked, chopped)
- Juice from ½ Lime
- ½ tsp Chili Powder
- 1 Garlic Clove (chopped)
- 2 Seeded Wraps (or Whole Grain Tortillas)
- 1 Avocado (halved, stoned)
- 1 Roasted Red Pepper (from jar)
- Olive Oil
- 1-2 Sprigs Cilantro (chopped)

Method

1. In a bowl, toss together chicken, garlic, chili powder, and lime juice. Heat 2 tablespoons oil in a pan over medium-high heat. Add chicken mixture and red pepper. Cook 1-2 minutes until warm.

2. Heat wraps (or tortillas) over a low flame on the stove until both sides just start to char. Divide avocado evenly into each wrap. Crush and spread with a fork. Divide chicken and pepper mixture evenly into each wrap. Sprinkle cilantro over the top. Roll and enjoy.

Health Facts

Avocado gets its uniquely silky texture from a combination of unsaturated fat and fiber making this the absolute perfect food to help fight cravings.

Chicken and whole grain wraps provide a good dose of protein to keep you powering through the day.

Garlic acts as a natural antibacterial and antiviral. So, add an extra clove or two if you feel a cold coming on!

33. Spinach & Egg Pizza

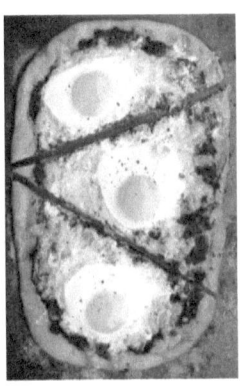

Pizza is upgraded from junk food to high-end meal in this recipe with fresh spinach and eggs.

Ingredients

- 2 Seeded Wraps (or Whole Grain Tortillas)
- Olive Oil
- 1 Roasted Red Pepper (from jar)
- 2 Tomatoes
- 2 Tbsps. Tomato Paste
- 1 Tbsp. Dill (chopped)
- 2 Tbsps. Parsley (chopped)
- 2 Eggs
- 1-2 handfuls Spinach
- ¼ cup Grated Mozzarella
- ½ Red Onion (thinly sliced)

Method

1. Preheat oven to 375°F. Lay wraps (or tortillas) on a baking sheet. Brush liberally with oil. Bake 3 minutes. Chop tomatoes and pepper. Stir together with tomato paste. Season with dill and parsley.

2. Turn tortillas oil-side down. Spread tomato mixture over them. Leave the center free of any large chunks of tomato or pepper. Sprinkle cheese on top.

3. Crack an egg into the center of each tortilla. Return to oven. Bake 10 minutes (or until egg white is cooked and egg is set). Sprinkle red onion and spinach over the top to serve.

Health Facts

Despite what you might have heard, eggs are actually a superfood. They help lower cholesterol and decrease blood pressure. So, eat up!

Spinach is a great source of vitamin K, calcium, iron, and magnesium making it one of the best foods for your bones and muscles. No wonder Popeye was chowing this down by the can-full!

The tomato and pepper spread provide you with a rich dose of lycopene and other key antioxidants.

34. Carrot & Lentil Soup

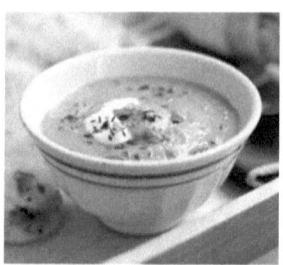

Carrot and lentil are married together in this creamy soup that truly soothes the soul.

Ingredients

- 1 Onion (thinly sliced)
- Olive Oil
- 3 Garlic Cloves (sliced)
- 2 Carrots (diced)
- ½ cup Red Lentils
- 1 Chicken Stock Cube (crumbled)
- 2 Tbsps. Parsley (chopped)

Method

1. Bring 1 ½ quarts of water to a boil in a pot over high heat. Heat 2 tablespoons oil in a pan over medium-high heat. Add onion. Cook 2 minutes. Add carrots and garlic. Cook 1 minute.

2. Add 1 quart of boiling water. Stir in crumbled stock cube and red lentils. Cover. Cook over medium heat 15 minutes (or until lentils are tender). Remove from heat. Stir in parsley. Divide into bowls. Serve with a dollop of plain Greek yogurt.

Health Facts

The high amount of vitamin A in this soup will help protect eyes, skin, hair, and nails.

Carrots are actually more nutritious when cooked because your body can digest the nutrients more easily.

Red lentils are a great source of both protein and fiber.

35. Tuna Stuffed Summer Squash

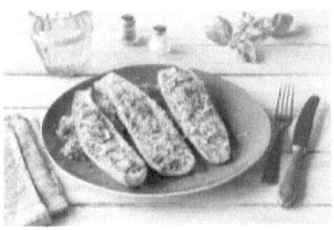

Summer squash gets a burst of juicy flavor with the addition of tuna and cottage cheese.

Ingredients

- 1 ½ cups canned Tuna (drained)
- 1 Red Chili (chopped)
- 1 Spring Onion (sliced)
- 1 handful Cherry Tomatoes (halved)
- ½ bunch Cilantro (chopped)
- 1 medium Squash
- 1 cup Cottage Cheese

Method

1. Preheat oven to 375°F. Poke squash repeatedly with a fork. Bake in oven for 1 hour (or until softened). In a bowl, mix together tuna, tomatoes, cilantro, spring onion, and chili. Slice squash in half. Remove seeds or create a hollow in the flesh. Fill with tuna mixture and cottage cheese. Serve.

Health Facts

With lots of veggies, this dish provides a healthy range of all vitamins and minerals.

Tuna is an excellent source of both protein and unsaturated fats.

Canned tuna is one of the most sustainable sources of this over-fished species.

36. Butternut Squash Salad

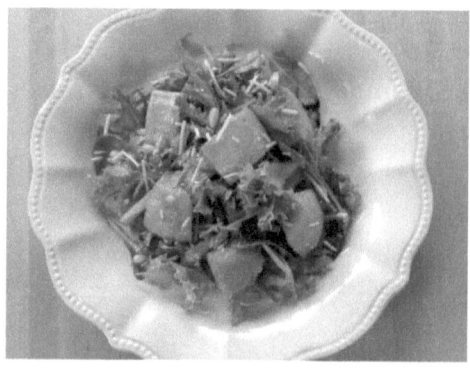

Butternut squash turns this salad into a hearty meal with rich flavor.

Ingredients

- 1 Butternut Squash (peeled, seeded, diced)
- Olive Oil
- 1/3 cup Brown Rice
- 1/3 cup Lentils
- 1 head Broccoli (chopped)
- 1/3 cup Dried Cranberries
- 1-2 handfuls Pumpkin Seeds
- Juice from 1 Lemon

Method

1. Preheat oven to 375°F. Arrange squash in a single layer on a baking sheet. Drizzle olive oil liberally over squash pieces. Bake 30 minutes or until softened. Submerge rice and lentils together in water until fully covered. Bring to a boil. Reduce heat. Simmer until water is absorbed and rice is fluffy.

2. Add broccoli just before rice is finished. Cook 4 minutes. Stir in cranberries and pumpkin seeds. Season to taste. Pour mixture into a bowl. Add squash. Pour in lemon juice. Toss to combine. Serve.

Health Facts

Butternut squash is a great source of beta-carotene which acts as a natural "sunscreen" in your skin by making it more resistant to UV rays.

The lentils and brown rice combine to make a complete protein.

Broccoli provides even more fiber along with plenty of essential minerals.

37. Tomato Chorizo Salad

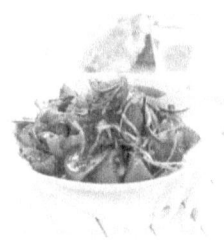

Tomato and chorizo combine for a wonderfully rich and complex flavor pallet in this simple and effortless salad. It's a meal in itself or a great side to the stuffed chicken breasts below.

Ingredients

- 3 large Tomatoes (cut into wedges)
- 1 Red Onion (thinly sliced)
- 2-3 sprigs Thyme (leaves removed, stems discarded)
- Sherry Vinegar
- Olive Oil
- 1 cup Chorizo (sliced)

Method

1. In a large bowl, combine tomatoes, onions, and thyme. Season to taste. Drizzle oil and vinegar and over (to taste). Set aside. Heat a dry pan over high heat. Cook chorizo slices until browned on both sides. Toss chorizo into tomato mixture. Pour some pan drippings. Toss to combine. Serve.

Health Facts

Tomatoes are one of the best sources of the antioxidant, lycopene and cooking them makes this antioxidant even more digestible.

Thyme is great for digestion and helps detox the body.

Olive oil is one of the healthiest sources of unsaturated fats. Don't be afraid to drizzle on a little extra!

38. Chicken Breasts Stuffed with Feta & Sundried Tomatoes

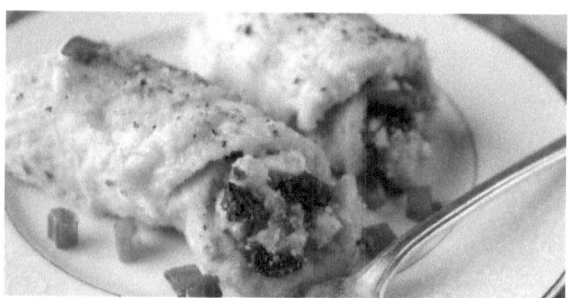

Your plain old pan-fried chicken dinner just got a whole lot more exciting with the simple addition of feta and sundried tomatoes.

Ingredients

- 1 Tbsp. Dried Tomatoes
- 4 Skinless Boneless Chicken Breasts
- ¼ cup Crumbled Feta Cheese
- 2 Tbsps. Cream Cheese
- 2 tsp Fresh Basil (crushed)
- 1/8 tsp Pepper
- Olive Oil
- 4 Fresh Basil Sprigs (to garnish)

Method

1. In a small bowl, combine tomatoes and boiling water (enough to submerge tomatoes). Let stand 10 minutes. Drain and pat tomatoes dry. Set aside. Slice a pocket into the center of each chicken breast. The slice should be made horizontally across the thickest part. Slice deeply but not through to the other side.

2. In a bowl, combine cream cheese, feta, basil, and tomatoes. Divide mixture evenly into each of the chicken breasts. Use toothpicks to close opening. Sprinkle breasts with pepper. Heat 3-4 tablespoons oil in a large pan over medium-high heat. Cook chicken 12-14 minutes or until cooked through (turning once). Reduce heat if chicken starts to brown too quickly. Divide onto plates. Garnish with a sprig of basil. Serve. Optional: serve on a bed of tomato quinoa (prepare quinoa according to package directions, adding 1 diced tomato, salt and pepper to taste).

Health Facts

Feta (and other goat cheeses) are the only cheese that naturally contains vitamin D!

Tomatoes are full of antioxidants which help protect your skin from sun damage.

Basil is great for digestion and helps treat bad breath!

39. Salmon on A Bed of Spinach, Pears & Blue Cheese

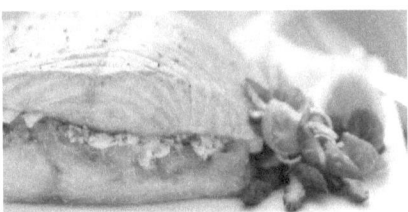

The delicate flavors of each ingredient are able to shine in this recipe. The boldness of the blue cheese ties it all together wonderfully.

Ingredients

- 2 large Salmon Fillets (about ½ lb. each)
- 1 tsp Dried Sage (crushed)

- Salt & Pepper to taste
- 4 Tbsps. Butter (divided)
- 6 oz. Baby Spinach
- 1 large Pear (cored, thinly sliced)
- ¼ cup Crumbled Blue Cheese

Method

1. Slice fillets in half to make 4 smaller fillets. Rub with sage, salt, and pepper. Heat 2 tablespoons butter in a large pan over medium-high heat. Sear salmon on all sides. It should still be cooked on the outside but still pink on the inside (about 8-10 minutes total).

2. Place salmon on plates. Add spinach to pan. Cook until just starting to wilt. Remove from pan onto plate. In a small pan over medium-high heat, melt remaining butter and cook pear slices. Cook 5 minutes, stirring occasionally. Pears should be soft and lightly browned. Divide spinach evenly onto 4 plates. Divide pear slices. Top with salmon fillets. Crumble blue cheese over. Serve. If blue cheese is too pungent, try feta instead.

Health Facts

Salmon is one of the best sources of healthy unsaturated fats which hydrate dry skin, even out skin tone, and strengthen brittle hair!

The spinach is full of iron and by lightly cooking it, you're making that iron even easier for your body to digest.

Cheese provides a protein boost along with calcium.

40. Chicken Walnut Berry Salad

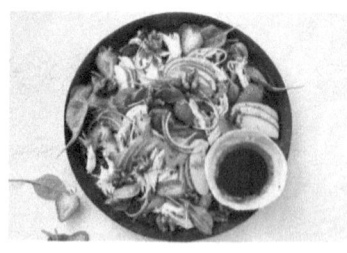

The combination of chicken, walnut, and berry in this salad create an exquisitely harmonious blend of flavors.

Ingredients

- Raspberry Vinegar
- Olive Oil
- 2 Tbsps. Fresh Mint (chopped)
- 2 Tbsps. Honey
- ¼ tsp Salt
- 4 cups Fresh Spinach
- 2 cups Chicken Breast (cooked, chopped)
- 2 cups Fresh Strawberries (sliced)
- ½ cup Fresh Blueberries
- ¼ cup Toasted Walnuts (chopped)
- ¼ cup Crumbled Goat Cheese
- ½ tsp Pepper

Method

1. In a sealable jar, combine ½ cup oil, ¼ cup vinegar, mint, honey, and salt. Seal jar. Shake vigorously. In a large bowl, mix together chicken, blueberries, strawberries, walnuts, cheese, and spinach. Toss to combine. Divide salad evenly among 4 plates. Shake dressing again. Drizzle over salads. Sprinkle with pepper. Serve.

Health Facts

Think of this salad as a superfood. It's full of everything you need.

If you eat this all to yourself (divided into a couple meals throughout the day), you'll get all 9 servings of fruits and veggies for the day!

Berries are rich in antioxidants which help detox your body and clear up blemished skin.

41. Lemon Pepper Tuna on A Bed of Veggie Couscous

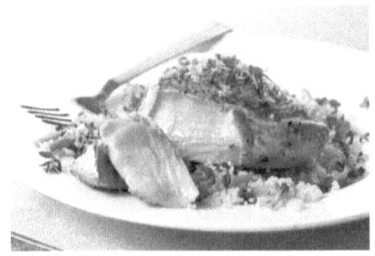

Lemon and pepper create the perfect balance between bold and delicate on these tuna steaks.

Ingredients

- 4 (1" thick) Tuna Steaks
- 2 Tbsps. Lemon Juice
- 1 tsp Low Sodium Soy Sauce
- 1 tsp Fresh Thyme (crushed)
- ½ tsp Lemon Pepper Seasoning
- 2 cups Broccoli (chopped)
- ½ cup Carrots (grated)
- 1 cup Chicken Broth
- 2/4 cup Water
- 2 Garlic Cloves (minced)
- 1 cup Whole Grain Couscous
- 1 Tbsp. Fresh Thyme Leaves
- Olive Oil

Method

1. In a small bowl, combine lemon juice, soy sauce, teaspoon thyme, and lemon pepper seasoning. Brush mixture over one side of each tuna steak.

2. Lightly grease the rack of the broiler pan with oil. Place tuna steaks (brushed side up) on rack. Broil 8-12 minutes or until fish becomes flakey (turning once and brushing other side with lemon mixture).

3. In a pot, bring water to a boil with chicken broth, carrot, broccoli, and garlic. Cover. Cook 3 minutes. Stir in couscous. Remove from heat. Let cool 5 minutes. Fluff couscous with a fork. Serve fish on top of couscous mixture. Garnish with thyme leaves.

Health Facts

Tuna is a superfood. It's packed with protein, vitamins and minerals.

It's also one of the best sources of Omega 3 Fatty Acids which are essential for heart and brain health.

The couscous helps provide a few of your daily servings of veggies.

42. Maple Pecan Pork Chops

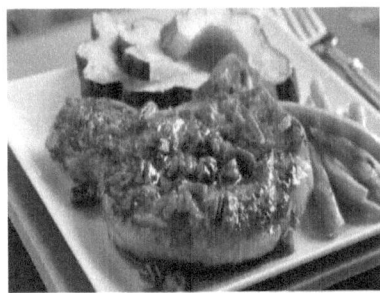

These pork chops pair perfectly with the butternut squash salad found in this book.

Ingredients

- 4 Boneless Pork Loin Chops (about ¾" thick)
- ¼ tsp Salt
- ¼ tsp Pepper
- Olive Oil
- 2 Tbsps. Shallot (finely chopped)
- 2 Tbsps. Toasted Pecans (chopped)
- 2 Tbsps. Maple Syrup
- 1 Tbsp. Melted Butter
- 1 Tbsp. Fresh Thyme (crushed)

Method

1. Sprinkle salt and pepper over each pork chop. In a large pan over medium-high heat, add 3-4 tablespoons olive oil. When hot, add shallots. Cook 1 minute, stirring constantly. Add pork chops. Cook 9-13 minutes, turning once. Pork juices should run clear.

2. In a small bowl, mix together syrup, butter, pecans, and thyme. Place pork chops onto serving plates. Drizzle over with syrup mixture. Serve alongside salad or quinoa.

Health Facts

Real maple syrup is a good substitute for refined sugar. It's full of minerals like manganese and potassium. Remember to get real maple syrup and not maple-flavored syrup!

The pecans and olive oil are providing you with a rich source of unsaturated fats which are great for losing weight and nourishing your skin.

Thyme is beneficial for digestion problems.

43. Healthy Whole Wheat and Oats Pumpkin Pancakes

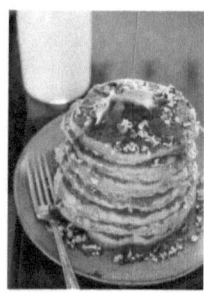

This healthy recipe for pancakes provides only 118 calories/81 grams. It is also a rich source of carbohydrates, fiber, proteins and a small amount of fat is also provided.

Buttermilk can be replaced by sour milk which can be easily made at home. Blend lemon juice or vinegar in 1 cup of nonfat milk. Set aside for 10 minutes before utilizing. For toppings roasted nuts can be used. Cook the nuts for 2 to 4 minutes in a small pan. The pan should be heated on medium flame. Stir till the nuts turn light brown.

Preparation time: 5 minutes
Total time: 5 minutes

Ingredients

- Eggs (3 big)
- Brown sugar (⅓ cup)
- Apple sauce (½ cup)
- Pumpkin puree (½ cup)
- Buttermilk (1½ cup)
- Vanilla extract (2 teaspoon)
- Whole wheat flour (1 cup)
- Rolled oats (1 cup)
- Baking powder (2 tablespoon)
- Salt (½ teaspoon)
- Pumpkin spice (1 teaspoon)

Method

1. Mix the eggs, buttermilk, brown sugar, apple sauce and pumpkin puree together in a large bowl. The batter should be well combined. Then add the flour, vanilla, salt, pumpkin spice, baking powder and the oats. Mix again thoroughly to obtain a perfect batter.

2. Take a scooped spoon and half fill it with the prepared batter. Pour it in a pan heated on medium heat. Cook for 3 minutes so that the sides become firm then cook the other side of the pancake for about 1 to 2 minutes. Sprinkle or spread maple syrup, butter or roasted pecans.

To store these pancakes, keep in refrigerator in an airtight container.

Did You Know?

Fresh pumpkin puree contains just 50 calories and no fat, is a rich source of vitamin A, vital for vision and immunity. It also contains fiber and potassium, two very important nutrients.

Pumpkins remind us of Halloween, and those bred for jack-o-lanterns have a larger seed cavity, longer stems, and thinner walls for easier carving, while pumpkins for eating tend to be smaller and more solid. The flat white seeds that you scoop out are the unhulled, milder-tasting version of the smaller green seeds, or pepitas found in stores, Enjoy the white seeds as a snack, and add pepitas to salads, soups, or granola.

44. Low-Fat and Healthy Buttermilk Waffles

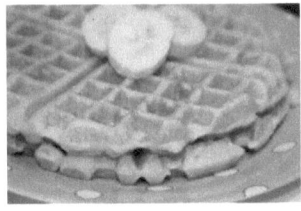

This waffle recipe is especially enjoyed by children and diet conscious people. It is easy to make and children also like making them. Each waffle only provides less than 100 calories, 3 g of fats and less than 15 g of carbohydrates.

Preparation time: 15 minutes
Cooking time: 10 minutes
Makes: 4 to 6 servings

Ingredients

- All-purpose flour (1 cup)
- Toasted wheat germ (2 tablespoons)
- Sugar (2 tablespoons)
- Baking powder (1 teaspoon)
- Baking soda (1/2 teaspoon)
- Salt (1/4 teaspoon)
- Nonfat or low-fat buttermilk (1 cup)
- Vegetable oil (1 tablespoon)
- Egg, lightly beaten (1 large)
- Cooking spray
- Maple syrup bananas (optional)

Method

1. In a measuring cup, mix flour, wheat germ, sugar, baking powder, baking soda and salt. In a separate bowl whisk oil, buttermilk and egg together. Add this mixture to the dry one and whip until incorporated.

2. Preheat a waffle iron after applying the cooking spray. Pour quarter of a cup on the hot waffle, spreading it evenly. Let it cook for about 3 to 5 minutes or until the lights tell you. These waffles can be served with either bananas or maple syrup.

This recipe will also work as pancakes. You may freeze leftover waffles by wrapping them tightly in foil and reheating them in a toaster oven.

45. Coconut Chocolate Energy Truffle Recipe

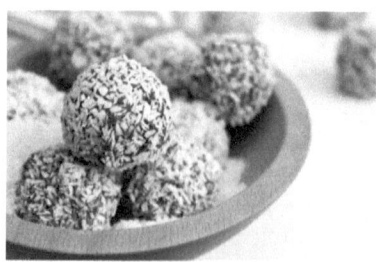

These creamy coconut-cocoa truffles, each one of them are fueled with revitalizing nutrients. These bite-sized snacks are powered by slow-burning natural sugars and protein. Have two truffles for your mid-afternoon snack, and you'll be fresh until dinnertime.

This recipe makes 40 truffles, with 92 calories per truffle, cooking time 45 minutes, total time 5-6 hours (including chill time)

Ingredients

For the truffles

- Coarsely chopped, pitted medjool dates-2 cups
- Boiling water-1 cup
- Raw almonds-1 cup
- Melted coconut oil-2 tablespoons
- Vanilla extract-1 teaspoon
- Sea salt-1/2 teaspoon
- Coconut flour
- Unsweetened cocoa powder 3/4 cup+3 tablespoons

For the chocolate coating

- Dark chocolate cut into small pieces (8 ounces-70% cacao content or higher)
- Coconut oil-2 tablespoons
- Boiling water-1/2 cup
- Unsweetened shredded coconut -1 cup

Method

1. Grind the almonds in a food processor until it turns into a creamy paste (for about 7 minutes). Add the dates and standing water, vanilla, coconut oil and salt to the processor. Blend until a smooth paste is formed, scraping down the sides a couple of times in between. Now put in the cocoa and coconut dough and process until a dough-like paste is formed. Refrigerate it for about 2-3 hours until very cold.

2. Line a baking tray with foil or parchment paper. Roll 40 balls out of the mixture using 1 tablespoon per truffle. Take coconut oil and chocolate in a heat-safe container. Add boiling water to it and mix gently with a spatula until the mixture becomes smooth.

3. With a fork dip each ball into the chocolate mixture and let the excess drip off. Prepare a separate tray of shredded coconut and roll the truffles to cover them fully. Transfer them to the prepared baking tray and refrigerate until the chocolate is set.

Did You Know?

Dates also known as nature's candy are a rich source of dietary fiber, iron and potassium. It is also a great source of B vitamins, which helps maintain energy levels. Almonds are one of the richest protein nuts, have satiating power and are high in monounsaturated fats and vitamin E.

46. Deep Dark Chocolate Layer Cake

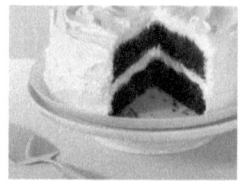

This deep dark chocolate layer cake makes 16 servings and provides 352 calories per slice. Also, it is low in fats and carbohydrates and contains almost no cholesterol. It is an ideal treat for people with a sweet tooth.

Ingredients

For the Cake

- Cooking spray
- All-purpose flour-3 cups
- Sugar-2 cups
- Sifted natural unsweetened cocoa powder-2/3 cup
- Baking soda-2 teaspoons
- Teaspoon salt-3/4
- Brewed coffee, at room temperature-1½ cups
- Canola oil-2/3 cup
- Egg whites-2 large
- Apple cider vinegar-2 tablespoons
- Vanilla extract-2 teaspoons

For the Frosting

- Egg whites-3 large
- Sugar-1½ cups
- Cream of tartar-1/4 teaspoon
- Dash of salt
- Vanilla extract-1 teaspoon

Method

1. Preheat oven to 350°F. Set a rack in the center of the oven; Apply cooking spray on 2 (9- x 1 1/2 -inch) round cake pans. Cover base of pans with parchment paper and spray with cooking oil; set it aside.

2. To prepare cake: Mix cocoa, flour, baking soda, sugar and salt in a big bowl, beating well. In another medium bowl, blend egg whites, vinegar, coffee, oil, and vanilla, mixing well. Incorporate coffee mixture into flour mixture, whisking until smooth. Separate batter uniformly between into the two ready pans; tap pan on a work surface to break air pockets.

3. Cook in the oven until a wooden toothpick placed in the center of the cakes comes out clean (around ½ hr. to 35 minutes.). Chill in pans on a wire rack for about 15-20 minutes. With a knife, loosen the edges of cakes by running it around the sides; turn cakes upside down onto a cooling frame. Take out the parchment; completely cool on rack.

4. To prepare frosting: Mix egg whites, cream of tartar, sugar and salt in a big deep heatproof bowl and set it over 1½ inches of bubbling water; whip with an electric blender at medium-high speed (about 7 minutes). Remove bowl from saucepan; keep on beating until totally chilled (about 3 minutes). Blend in vanilla.

5. Carefully position 1 cake layer on a plate. Using a spatula spread a layer of frosting over it; now place the remaining cake. Evenly spread left over frosting over top and sides of complete cake.

Unsweetened cocoa powder, egg whites and coffee, lightens up this fluffy favorite.

47. Low Fat Strawberry Cheesecake

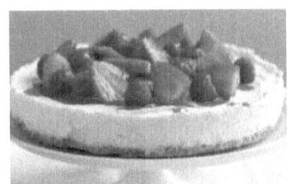

Serves: 8
Chill Time: 3 Hr.
Cook Time: 35 Min

The next time someone tells you they're coming over, ask if they'd rather have a low-fat sweet dish or cheesecake. Of course, with this one you'll get the best of both slices after slice!

Ingredients

- 1% low-fat cottage cheese-16 ounces
- Egg substitute*-3/4 cup
- Reduced-fat cream cheese 4 ounces-softened
- Sugar-1/3 cup+1 tablespoon (divided)
- Vanilla extract-1 teaspoon
- Low-fat vanilla yogurt-1/2 cup
- Lemon juice-1/8 teaspoon
- Sliced fresh strawberries-1 pint

Method

1. Preheat oven to 350°F. Coat a 9" pie plate with cooking spray. Combine cream cheese, cottage cheese, egg substitute, 1/3 cup sugar, and vanilla in a blender for 1 minute, until smooth. Pour into the prepared 9-inch pie plate. Bake for about half an hour to 40 minutes, or until the center is firm.

2. In a small bowl, combine remaining yogurt, 1 tablespoon sugar, and lemon juice and blend well. Spread uniformly over cheesecake, and then bake for 5 minutes. Take out from oven and cool entirely. Top with sliced strawberries, then cover loosely and chill for at least 3 hours prior to serving.

Other toppings include a combination of blackberries, raspberries, and blueberries, or even sliced kiwifruit!

48. Creamy Cheese Chocolate Chip Cookies

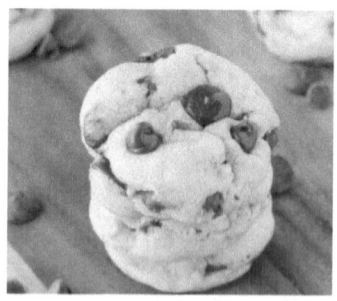

Makes about 10-12

A holiday becomes a reason to eat more cookies and these tempting cheese cream cookies are some of the most delicious, lightest, softest, chewiest cookies ever to come out of the kitchen…Yet have just 40 calories… and less than 2 grams of fat each! Try and stop at just one.

Ingredients

- 1/3 cup+1/4 cup oat flour OR
- Salt-1/8 tsp.
- Baking soda-1/4 tsp.
- Dark chocolate chips 2-5 tbsp., or as desired
- Sugar granules or xylitol 1/4 cup (46g)
- Cream cheese(full-fat), such as Tofutti-3 tbsp. (45g)
- Pure vanilla extract-1/2 tsp.
- Melted coconut oil-1 tbsp. (12g)

Method

1. In a deep bowl, combine the first 5 ingredients. In a cup, beat together the remaining 3 ingredients. If the cheese is too firm heat it a little so that it blends. Pour the wet ingredients into the dry, then mix together and do not include extra liquid. Keep stirring and scraping off the spoon as you whip till it forms a smooth batter.

2. Shape into a big ball, then shape it into cookie dough balls and freeze for at least half an hour on a plate. Preheat oven to 325 F and grease a cookie tray, when ready to bake. Bake for 8 minutes—they will seem quite undercooked when they come out, wait for at least 10 minutes by which time they should harden.

Fun Fact

Cocoa and dark chocolate have many health benefits; they contain a large amount of antioxidants (flavonoids) which may assist in keeping high blood pressure down and lessen the risk of stroke and heart attacks. The darker the chocolate, the more beneficial it is. According to an Italian study, a small square (20g) of dark (bittersweet) chocolate every three days is the ideal dose for cardiovascular benefits. Eating more does not offer added benefits.

49. Low-Cal, Low-Fat Mashed Potatoes with Crispy Golden Chicken

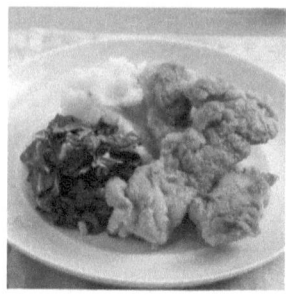

This is a low fat and low calorie (per 2/3-cup serving: 156 calories, 34g carbohydrate) version of the popular classic side dish.

To avoid an overload on carbohydrates, try adding cauliflower or some beans that are lower in carbs and have much higher protein content (and antioxidants) to give the consistency of classic mashed potatoes.

Yields: 6 servings
Preparation time: 20 minutes
Cooking time: 35 minutes

Ingredients

- Garlic cloves 8 to 10
- Quartered potatoes, 2 pounds (Yukon Gold recommended)
- Light sour cream 1/3 cup
- Fat-free milk 1/4 cup
- Shredded fresh rosemary, oregano, or thyme-1 tablespoon
- Salt 1/2 teaspoon
- Black pepper 1/4 teaspoon

Method

1. **To roast garlic:** wrap unpeeled cloves in foil, bake at 400°F for about half an hour or until cloves feel squashy when pressed. Squeeze garlic from peels into a small bowl when cool enough.

2. Meanwhile, dip the potatoes in cold water a large saucepan and bring to a boil over high heat. Cook the potatoes on low heat or until tender, for about 20 minutes. Remove the potatoes and peel them. With a potato masher or an electric mixer (on low speed), mash potatoes and

garlic. Add milk, sour cream; herbs-oregano, rosemary, or thyme; salt; and black pepper. Whip until soft and fluffy.

Healthy Cooking Tips

The potatoes may become mushy if you directly place the potatoes in hot/warm water for boiling, the cold ingredients like milk and sour cream should be a room temperature before adding it to the hot potatoes. Do not over mix the ingredients.

The roasted garlic and the fresh herbs add a rich flavor to the potatoes, help in reducing cholesterol, and the low-fat sour cream gives a silky consistency and a dash of flavor.

50. Crispy Golden Chicken

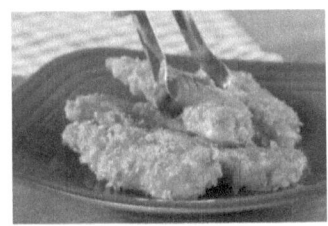

Serves: 8
Preparation Time: 5 min
Cooking Time: 20 min

Chicken is a good source of protein, trim off the fat and prefer chicken breasts to legs or thighs as they contain less fat

Ingredients

- 2 beaten egg whites,
- Almond flour-1 cup (150 g)
- Paprika-1 tsp.
- Garlic powder-1 tsp.
- Salt-1/2 tsp.
- Black pepper-1/2 tsp.
- Dried thyme-1/2 tsp.
- Chipotle powder-1 tsp. (optional)
- Chicken breast tenders-2 pounds (900 g), rinsed and patted dry
- 2-4 tablespoon olive oil

Method

1. Whisk egg whites in a shallow dish. In another medium sized bowl, combine all dry ingredients, and mix well. Dip chicken in the beaten eggs mixture. And then cover it in the dry mixture. In a medium sized skillet, heat oil and place the chicken in it and allow both sides to brown (about 3-4 minutes each side).

Cooking tip

If you want crispier and very well-done chicken, place the fried pieces on a sheet pan in such a way that there is space between the pieces. Put chicken in oven for 10-15 minutes. Remove and serve.

51. Chicken Breasts Stuffed with Pimiento Cheese

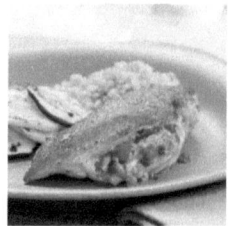

Filling skinless boneless, chicken breasts with scallions, pimientos and cheese gives them grand taste effortlessly. Don't be worried if some of the stuffing falls out while the chicken is baking; just scoop it up from the pan as you dish out. Serve with: Sautéed summer squash or zucchini and barley. It is an extremely nutritious dish with just 200 calories per serving, low in cholesterol, fats and carbohydrates. This recipe makes 4 servings and requires just 45 minutes in preparation.

Ingredients

- Gouda cheese, preferably smoked and shredded (1/2 cup)
- Chopped scallion/green spring onions (2 tablespoons)
- Sliced pimientos, chopped (1 tablespoon)
- Paprika, divided (1 teaspoon)
- Chicken breasts 4 small boneless, skinless trimmed and tenders removed (total 1¼-1½ pounds)
- Salt (1/2 teaspoon divided)
- Freshly ground pepper, divided (1/2 teaspoon)
- Extra-virgin olive oil (1 tablespoon)

Method

1. Heat oven to 400 degrees. In a small bowl, mix pimientos, Gouda, scallion and ½ teaspoon paprika. Cut a slit in the side of the chicken length wise so that it opens like a book. Season the inside with salt and pepper. Dividing the cheese equally among the breasts, press the block of cheese and close the chicken. Then rub the remaining salt, pepper and paprika on the outside of the chicken breasts.

2. Place the seasoned chicken in hot oil over medium heat. Cook for about 2 minutes until one side turns golden brown. Then flip the chicken on the other side, turn off the heat and place the cooking pan in the oven. Let it bake until the chicken is not pink. To check if the chicken is well cooked insert an instant read thermometer in the inner of the chicken. If the thermometer reads 165 degrees or above then your chicken is perfect.

Tips & notes

If a small breast is not available take off the tenders of a 5 to 6-ounce chicken breast. The tenders can be frozen and later be stir-fried. You can add other ingredients to the stuffing inside the chicken for example mushrooms, broccoli and onions. It gives a unique taste and is more filling.

52. Black Bean and Quinoa Burgers

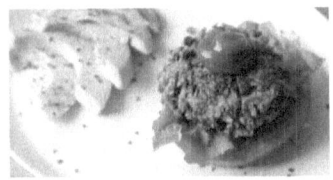

For more frequent burger urges, try something a tad healthier to overcome the craving. These black bean and quinoa burgers are packed with protein and fiber which leads to efficient digestion and a healthy heart.

Toss these patties on a lettuce bun with avocado and a dollop of homemade ketchup, some chopped sliced tomato and it's a winning burger for both taste and nutrition! Place a slice of sharp cheddar if you're feeling indulgent.

Ingredients

- (15.5 ounces) black beans, rinsed and drained-1 can
- Cooked quinoa-1/2 cup

- Cumin- 1/2 teaspoon
- Freshly ground black pepper-1/2 teaspoon
- Paprika-1/2 teaspoon
- Sea salt1/2 teaspoon
- Nutritional yeast 1 tablespoon
- Extra-virgin olive oil (1 tablespoon) plus more for cooking

Method

1. Heat the oven to 400 degrees. Mash the beans in a bowl and mix well. The beans should be so well mashed that it is easy to shape into patties. Then make four equal patties. The ideal thickness for the patties is ¼ to ½ inch.

2. In an oven friendly dish heat ½ tablespoon olive oil on high heat and cook each side of patties in the oil for 1 minute or until light golden brown. Place the dish in the oven and cook for quarter of an hour. After that remove dish from oven and enjoy with either fresh buns or green vegetables with any topping you desire.

Facts

Quinoa contains 8 grams/1 cup serving of protein when cooked. Quinoa is an excellent alternate for rice and it's adaptable enough to make muffins, cookies, and breakfast dishes. It is packed with manganese, iron, fiber and magnesium. It is a unique plant based source of complete protein since it is totally gluten free.

53. Creamy Tarragon Chicken Salad

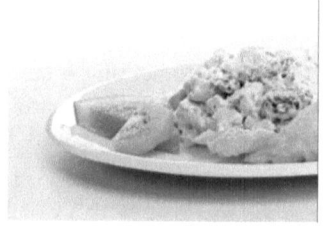

Ingredients

- Boneless, skinless chicken breast, trimmed (2 pounds)
- Reduced-sodium chicken broth (1 cup)
- Walnuts, chopped (1/3 cup)

- Reduced-fat sour cream (2/3 cup)
- Low-fat mayonnaise (1/2 cup)
- Dried tarragon (1 tablespoon)
- Salt (1/2 teaspoon)
- Freshly ground pepper (1/2 teaspoon)
- Diced celery (1 1/2 cups)
- Halved red seedless grapes (1 1/2 cups)

Method

1. Heat oven to about 450 degrees Fahrenheit. In a baking dish, place the chicken, making sure the chicken is evenly spread. Pour the broth and place in the oven for 30 to 35 minutes until the chicken center is not pinkish in color which can be checked by the instant read thermometer. After taking out the chicken from the oven, place it on the cutting board and leave it to cool down until it is cool enough to touch. Then dice it.

2. In the meantime, toast the walnuts in the oven, spread out on a baking tray, until fragrant and light golden. Then let them cool. Mix mayonnaise, sour cream, salt, pepper and tarragon in a large container or bowl. Add in the walnuts, chicken and grapes and turn and mix to cover well.

Tips & Notes

You can make the chicken beforehand to save time. The chicken can be baked and refrigerated for up to 2 days. The salad can be kept chilled for up to a day and include the nuts just prior to serving.

54. Fish and Chips with Tartar Sauce

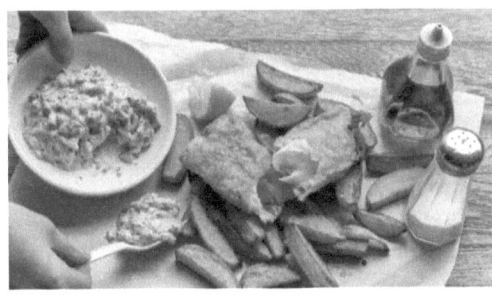

Serves: 4

Ingredients

For the Fish and Chips

- Fat-free buttermilk-3/4cup
- Fish fillets (catfish, tilapia, red snapper or your choice of firm fish fillets) 4(6 ounce)
- Potatoes, scrubbed and cut into sticks-1½lbs
- Paprika-3/4teaspoon
- Salt-½teaspoon
- Pepper-½teaspoon
- Cornmeal-2/3cup
- Old Bay Seasoning-½teaspoon
- Egg whites-2

For the tartar sauce

- Fat-free mayonnaise-1/3cup
- Scallion, chopped-1tablespoon
- Unsweetened pickle, chopped-1tablespoon
- Lemon juice-1teaspoon

Method

1. Add the fish into the buttermilk in a marinating dish or zip-lock bag, and mix well so that the fish is coated. Place the dish/bag in the refrigerator and keep for at least half an hour or up to 2 hours, turning the fish occasionally. Keep oven ready at 425° F. Cover with foil, two rimmed cookie sheets, inserting a rack in one of the pans. In the second pan, spray olive oil and spread potatoes evenly, sprinkle them with salt, paprika, and pepper; turn to coat. Cook the potatoes in the oven for half an hour.

2. On a sheet of wax paper or in a pie pan, blend together Old Bay Seasoning, the cornmeal and the remaining spices (1/4 tsp. each of paprika, salt and pepper) while the potatoes are baking. In another bowl, whisk egg whites until frothy. Discard the buttermilk and take out the fish fillets. Coat both sides of the fish in egg whites, and then in the cornmeal mixture, shaking off excess.

3. Place the fish onto a clean sheet of wax paper or a plate. Spray olive oil on both sides of fish and then place fish evenly in the pan on top of the rack. Bake fish for about 15 minutes or until done golden brown.

Simply combine the mayonnaise, pickle, scallion, and lemon juice, in a small bowl. While the fish and potatoes are cooking. Serve fish hot with tartar sauce and potatoes.

55. Roasted Red Pepper, Hummus, Avocado & Feta Sandwich

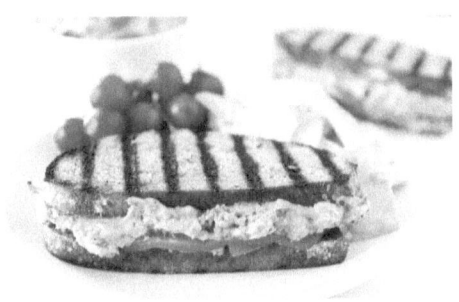

Makes: 2 sandwiches
Preparation Time: 5 minutes
Cooking Time: 10 minutes
Total Time: 15 minutes

This recipe is very flavorful and healthy. Its main ingredients are hummus, red pepper, feta cheese and avocado. The best part about this recipe is that it is less time consuming and easy to make.

Ingredients

- Whole wheat bread (4 slices)
- Hummus* (1/2 cup)
- Ripe (pit less) avocados (2)
- Crumbled feta cheese (1/4 cup)
- Fresh lemon juice (2 teaspoons)
- Freshly chopped basil (1 tablespoon)
- Salt and black pepper (to taste)
- Roasted red peppers, drained (1/2 cup)

Method

1. Spread the hummus smoothly on the bread and keep aside. Using a fork mash the avocado and feta cheese in a bowl. Then mix in the basil and lemon juice. Season with salt and pepper.

2. Now spread this mixture over the bread with the hummus. Then add toasted red pepper and place the other slice of bread to make the

sandwich. Spread a bit of oil or butter on the outer sides of the bread and toast it in a pan for 2 to 3 minutes. It can also be enjoyed without toasting.

Tip

Along with red peppers thinly sliced kalamata olives, cucumbers and red onions can also be used. Included here is the recipe of the Low-fat Hummus.

*Low-fat Spicy Hummus

This recipe of hummus provides 35.4 calories. It also provides sodium, proteins, fiber and good fats. It has no cholesterol and is low in carbohydrates.

Ingredients

- Low-sodium garbanzo beans, drained (15.5-ounce can)
- Fresh, squeezed lemon (1/2)
- Plain, fat-free yogurt (2 tablespoon)
- Fresh, peeled garlic (3-5 cloves)
- Salt (1/2 teaspoon)
- Water (1/4 cup)
- Cayenne Pepper (1 tablespoon)
- Light olive oil (1 tablespoon)

Method

1. Heat the garlic in a microwave until they tenderize or for about 30 to 40 seconds. Wash the garbanzo beans and then add all the other items in the blender. Course until all is well combined. The bean liquid can be used instead of olive oil to make the hummus less fatty. To reduce the amount of sodium you can exclude the salt and wash the beans thoroughly.

56. Mom's Easy Healthy Baked Beans

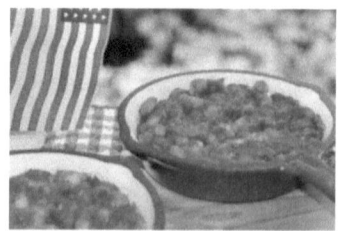

Mom's Healthy Baked Beans Secret Smokey Ingredient: This recipe's specialty is the liquid smoke which provides zero fats and a great taste to your food. The colgin or liquid smoke is a combination of vinegar, water, molasses, salt and a few other ingredients. Liquid smoke is also available in apple and pecan flavor

Serves: 8

Ingredients

- Virgin olive oil (2 tablespoons)
- Onions, finely chopped (2 cups)
- Salt (to taste)
- Organic tomato sauce (2 small cans)
- Organic Worcestershire sauce (1 tablespoon + 1 teaspoon)
- Liquid smoke (Hickory Flavor 4 tablespoons)
- Mustard (¾ teaspoon)
- Pure maple syrup (3 tablespoons)
- Cannellini beans, rinsed and drained (2 cans)

Method

1. Heat oven to about 325°F. Sauté onions in heated oil over medium flame for 5 to 6 minutes. Sprinkle salt over it for taste. Add the rest of the ingredients in the prepared onions and cook for another 5 minutes. Season to taste. Put the beans in a baking dish. Let the beans bake for 50 minutes.

Note

Beans are rich sources of protein, fiber and minerals. They are filling and will keep you satiated for long. Even though molasses has high carbohydrate content, you need not worry about that since the other ingredients balance out its effect being low in carbohydrates.

57. Quick Fall Minestrone

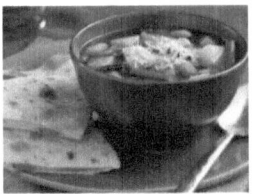

This recipe is a scrumptious meal made up of butternut squash and kale most enjoyed in the fall. This vegetarian soup is further made tastier and filling by adding beans and pasta.

Nutritional Information: This recipe provides proteins, fibers, sodium, calcium, iron and carbohydrates. It is also low in fats, cholesterol and provides only 212 calories

Ingredients

- Vegetable oil (1 tablespoon)
- Chopped onion (1 cup)
- Minced garlic (2 cloves)
- Vegetable broth (6 cups)
- Cubed peeled butternut squash (2 1/2 cups)
- Cubed peeled baking potato (2 1/2 cups)
- Cut green beans (1 cup)
- Diced carrot (1/2 cup)
- Dried oregano (1 teaspoon)
- Freshly ground black pepper (1/2 teaspoon)
- Salt (1/4 teaspoon)
- Chopped kale (4 cups)
- Uncooked orzo (1/2 cup)
- Cannellini beans or other white beans, rinsed and drained (1 16-ounce can)
- Grated fresh Parmesan cheese (1/2 cup)

Method

1. In a pan, heat oil and sauté the garlic and onion over medium heat for about 2 to 3 minutes until it softens. Then add the other ingredients except for kale, orzo, beans and cheese into the pan and cook until it comes to a boil. Then lower the flames and keep stirring for 3 minutes. Then mix in the beans, kale and orzo and cook for a further 5 minutes. Top the grated cheese over it.

58. Healthier World's Best Lasagna

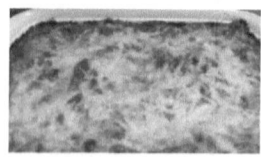

This low calorie and scrumptious recipe is really wholesome and healthy. It is another way for diet conscious people to enjoy their favorite meals. It is also a high protein recipe. To make it low fat, the parmesan cheese and salt have been left out.

Ingredients

- Lean ground turkey-1½ pound
- Minced onion-1/2 cup
- Crushed garlic,4 cloves
- 1 can crushed tomatoes-(28 ounce)
- Tomato paste-1can (6 ounce)
- Water-1/2 cup
- Dried basil leaves-1 teaspoon
- Fennel seeds-1/2 teaspoon
- Italian seasoning-1 teaspoon
- Ground black pepper-1/4 teaspoon
- Chopped fresh parsley-2 tablespoons
- Lasagna noodles-8
- 1 (8 ounce) fat-free ricotta cheese
- 1 (6 ounce) package shredded part-skim mozzarella cheese, divided

Method

1. Heat a large frying pan or Dutch oven over medium heat; cook for about 15 minutes and stir, ground turkey, garlic and onion, until well browned. Blend in tomato paste, crushed tomatoes, and water. Season with Italian seasoning, basil, fennel seeds, pepper, and 2 tablespoons parsley. Simmer for about 1½ hours, uncovered, stirring occasionally. Keep oven ready at 375°F (190°C). Bring to boil a large pot of lightly salted water. Cook lasagna in the boiling water, stirring seldom until cooked but stiff to bite, for about 8 minutes. Drain out the water.

2. Spread 1½ cups turkey sauce in the bottom of a baking dish. Arrange 4 noodles lengthwise over sauce. Spread the ricotta over noodles. Top with half of the mozzarella cheese. Spoon 1½ cups turkey sauce over mozzarella. Envelop with aluminum foil; make certain foil does not come in contact with the cheese to avoid sticking. Bake in preheated oven until sauce is hot and cheese has melted, about 25 minutes more. Remove foil and bake until cheese is golden brown, about 25 minutes. Cool for 15 minutes before serving.

Cooking tip

You can also add butternut squash, fresh spinach, or zucchini for added flavor.

59. Low-Calorie Cauliflower Crust Pizza (Gluten Free)

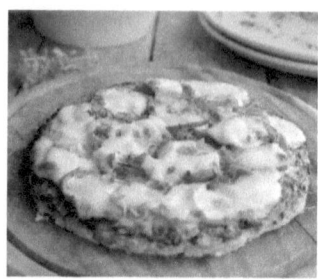

This pizza recipe is far healthier than the restaurant pizzas and is also appetizing. It comprises of a delicious wheat, tortilla and cauliflower crust topped with yummy vegetables and cheese. Be creative and make a flavorful pizza. It also provides a good amount of proteins and fiber which is very useful for the proper functioning of the heart.

Ingredients

- Raw cauliflower, fresh or frozen (340g)
- Egg (1 large)
- Low-fat mozzarella cheese, grate 50g and slice the remaining 25g for the topping (75g)
- Finely grated Parmesan cheese (2 tablespoons)
- Dried basil (1/4 teaspoon)
- Dried oregano (1/4 teaspoon)
- Garlic granules or powder (1/4 teaspoon)
- Salt (to taste)
- Fresh black pepper (to taste)
- Fresh tomatoes, thinly sliced (2)
- Red onion, peeled and thinly sliced (1/2)
- Fresh garlic, peeled and minced (2 cloves)
- Red chili flakes (1/4 teaspoon)
- Fresh oregano or basil (to garnish)

Method

1. Line a pizza tray with parchment paper. Heat oven to 210 degrees. Grate the cauliflower or process in a blender to obtain fine crumbs.

But take care not to make it in a puree. To soften the cauliflower crumbs, microwave it for at least 5 to 6 minutes. Add the egg, parmesan cheese, salt, cauliflower crumbs, mozzarella cheese, herbs, garlic powder and pepper in a bowl. Mix thoroughly until incorporated.

2. Flatten the dough in a 12.5cm large circle with 1.5cm thickness. Brush oil over it and bake it in the oven for 15 to 20 minutes or until golden brown. Then top the pizza crust with tomatoes, chili flakes, onion and garlic. Then cover it all with the cheese. Keep the pizza in the oven and let it bake for 10 minutes until the cheese has completely melted and the topping are cooked well. Sprinkle oregano or basil as seasoning.

Note

This pizza recipe is a low calorie one and suitable for people on Paleo diet and is also a vegan recipe. Each slice contains 240 calories and is very filling and tasty to eat.

60. Squash and Tomato Casserole

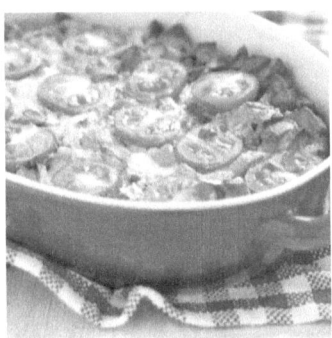

Few things are more calming than an enormous bowl of pasta with marinara sauce. But that means a lot of carbs? This "pasta" casserole substitutes the classic pasta with waistline-friendly spaghetti squash to fill those cravings without the extra calories and carbs. For the perfect healthy comfort food dinner, serve with a salad.

Ingredients

- Spaghetti squash-1
- Large carrots, diced-2
- Large yellow onion, diced-1

- (28oz) crushed tomatoes-1 large can
- Basil (dried or fresh)-1 teaspoon
- Dried oregano-½ teaspoon
- Garlic, chopped-3 cloves
- Low-fat or part-skim mozzarella, grated-¼ pound
- Extra-virgin olive oil-2 tablespoons
- Grated Parmesan cheese-½ cup (optional)

Method

1. Slice squash laterally and put it in a baking dish filled with 1 inch of water making the skin face down. Preheat the oven at 350 degrees and cover the dish with a foil and cook for about 45 minutes, making sure the squash is tender.

2. In the meantime, sauté the carrots and onion in hot olive oil for 10 minutes. Then sprinkle salt and pepper for flavor. Cook basil, oregano, garlic, crushed tomatoes and the prepared vegetables in an open vessel for quarter of an hour.

3. While the sauce is cooking take out the squash from the oven and let it cool enough so that it can be easily handled. Take out the seeds. Using a fork scrape the flesh. If the flesh comes off like spaghetti then you squash is well baked.

4. Now add the squash to the sauce that was cooking and turn off the stove mix all ingredients together. Then start layering the squash mixture and cheese alternately. First add squash mixture and then cheese and keep doing this until 8he sauce has finished.

5. Place the dish in the oven for at least half an hour, making sure the cheese is well melted. Set aside for about 15 to 20 minutes to let it cool and set completely.

Note

The flesh of spaghetti squash comes out in long threads, very much akin to the noodles for which it is called. In this recipe, the 'noodles' are thrown with vegetables and feta cheese. You can use a variety of vegetables, but be certain to use ones that have contrasting colors."

Grating the mozzarella cheese would be easier if it is frozen for 10 to 20 minutes.

61. Mom's Creamy Chicken and Broccoli Casserole

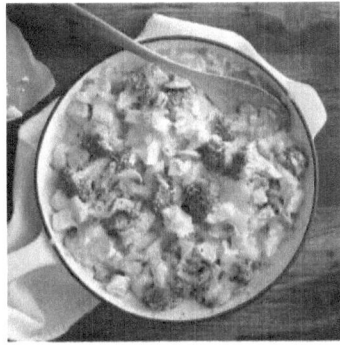

This recipe of creamy chicken provides less calories compared to the traditional one. It is lighter and also a yummy way of staying healthy and fit.

Nutritional Information: This dish provides only 277 calories and is also a great source of proteins, carbohydrates and fiber. It provides sodium, calcium and iron. It is low in fats and cholesterol.

Ingredients

- Steam-in-bag broccoli florets (1 12-ounce package)
- Canola oil (1 tablespoon)
- Already chopped onion (1 cup)
- Pre- sliced mushrooms (2 8-ounce packages)
- All-purpose flour (3 tablespoons)
- Fat-free milk (1 1/2 cups)
- Chopped skinless, boneless rotisserie chicken breast (about 3 cups)
- Plain fat-free Greek yogurt (1/2 cup)
- Canola mayonnaise (1/4 cup)
- Freshly ground black pepper (1/2 teaspoon)
- Salt (1/4 teaspoon)
- Sharp cheddar cheese, shredded (about 1/2 cup)
- Parmesan cheese, grated (about 1/4 cup)

Method

1. Heat the broiler. Microwave broccoli according to the instruction given on the package. Heat oil in a skillet on medium heat. Spread the oil and then put in the onions and mushrooms. Cook for about 10 to 12 minutes until the mushrooms turn brown, taking care not to burn it.

2. Then sprinkle flour over the prepared mixture and keep stirring for a minute. Then add the milk and stir until it boils. Cook for 3 minutes until it becomes of a thicker consistency. Put in the chicken and broccoli and cook for a further 1 minute. Then turn off the heat and mix in the salt, pepper, yoghurt and mayonnaise. Evenly spread the cheese and then let it broil for about 2 to 3 minutes.

62. Ground Beef and Texas Bean Enchiladas

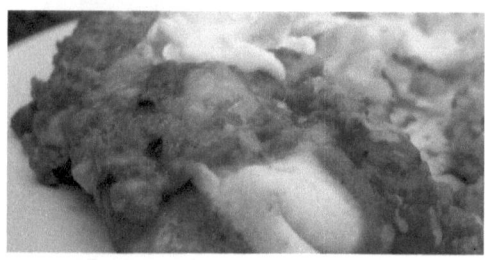

Preparation time: 20 minutes
Cooking time: 20 minutes
Total time: 40 minutes

This recipe is a remake of the traditional one. It is easy to make and is simple.

Ingredients

- Ground beef (1 pound)
- Pinto beans or black beans or Texas ranch style
- Beans (1 15 ounces can)
- Drained diced tomatoes (1 14 ounces can)
- Finely diced fresh poblano peppers (1/2 cup) or diced green chilies (1 4 ounces can)
- Finely diced white onions (1/2 cup)
- Crushed garlic (2 cloves)
- Shredded Mexican blend cheese or Monterey Jack Cheese (1 cup)
- Salt and pepper (to taste)
- (12 -15 8-inch) flour tortillas or whole wheat
- Flour tortillas or corn tortillas

For the Enchilada Sauce

- Hot water (2 1/4 cups)
- Tomato paste (1 6 ounces can)
- Margarine or butter (2 tablespoons)

- Flour (2 tablespoons)
- Red chili powder (5 teaspoons)
- Cumin (1 teaspoon)
- Garlic powder (2 teaspoons)
- Salt and pepper (to taste)

Method

1. Heat oven to 350 degrees. In a skillet mix onion, garlic, salt, pepper and ground beef. Cook until beef turns brown. Then let the grease drain. Then put in the canned chilies, peppers, beans of your choice and tomatoes in the skillet. Lower the heat, cover the dish and stir occasionally. In the meanwhile, prepare the sauce. Add all the ingredients required to make the sauce in a bowl and whip until all is completely combined. Then sprinkle the salt and pepper. Transfer ½ cup of sauce in the prepared meat mix. Then quickly turn off the heat. Coat each tortilla in the prepared sauce making sure it is completely covered.

2. In a pan place the sauce covered tortillas. Then put the meat mixture on one side of it and roll it. After rolling make sure that the open side is on the bottom so that the contents do not spill. Any remaining mixtures can be spread over the enchiladas. Wrap in foil and let it bake for 15 minutes. After removing the enchiladas from the oven, open the foil and evenly top with grated cheese. Put it in the oven again for 5 minutes so that the cheese melts. Cut the enchiladas into half and serve with either guacamole or rice or sour cream.

63. Low Salt, Low Fat Turkey Sloppy Joes

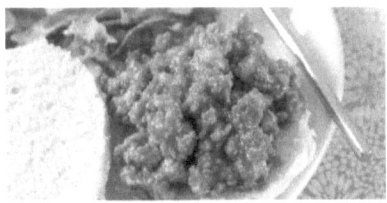

Serves: 6
Makes: 4 Sandwiches

Ingredients

- Lean ground turkey (1 pound)
- Onion (2/3 cup)

- Green pepper (1/2 cup)
- Jalapeno peppers (2)
- No-salt-added ketchup (1 cup)
- Brown sugar (2 tablespoons)
- Worcestershire sauce (2 tablespoons)
- Garlic powder (1 tablespoon)
- Chili powder (2 tablespoons)
- Mustard powder (1 tablespoon)
- Salt (1/4 teaspoon)
- Extra virgin olive oil (2 tablespoons)

Method

1. Dice the jalapenos after removing the seeds inside it. Also chop the onions and green pepper finely. Sauté the chopped items in a pan and keep aside. Then cook the turkey and drain it. In a pan over medium heat stir in all the ingredients for 3 to 5 minutes. Lower the heat and let it simmer for 8-10 minutes so that the flavors blend well. You can serve it on crusty rolls or any kind of bread you prefer.

Cooking tips

If you do not want it too hot, cut down the jalapenos or add more according to taste. Also, you may reduce the amount of brown sugar and try adding diced tomatoes and olives if you wish.

64. Sweet Potato Hash Browns

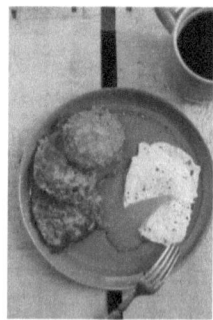

A traditional American comfort food to lift you out of any bad mood and warm you up completely

Serves: 2

Ingredients

- 1 pound diced sweet potatoes
- 3 tablespoon virgin olive oil
- 1 small onion, chopped
- 1 tablespoon chopped fresh parsley
- Salt and ground pepper

Method

1. Boil potatoes in salted water until tender but still firm to the touch. Rinse under cold water before chilling thoroughly. Heat 1 tablespoon oil in a pan over medium heat and sauté onions until soft and browned then set aside.

2. Add remaining oil to pan and add potatoes and stir as they cook until slightly browned. Add onions and allow to cook for a minute before tossing in parsley. Add seasoning and serve

Did You Know?

Allowing the potatoes to chill after they are boiled averts disintegration when they are sautéed

65. Curried Butternut Squash Bisque

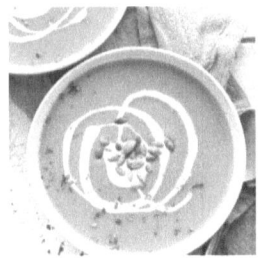

This creamy non-dairy soup allows you to eat clean and is a comforting meal that you can make in the comfort of your home. Great taste with no guilt attached.

Ingredients

- 1 teaspoon vegetable oil
- 1 chopped onion
- 2 minced cloves of garlic

- 3 cups peeled and chunked butternut
- 2 teaspoons curry paste
- 2 ½ cups water
- ½ cup coconut milk
- Salt to taste

Method

1. Heat oil over medium heat and sauté onion and garlic for twelve minutes. Add curry paste and sauté for a minute more. Add water and the butternut and allow to boil before reducing the heat. Cover pot and simmer until butternut is soft. Place mixture in blender and blend until smooth. Pour in the coconut milk then blend it in until mixture looks creamy. Put back into original pot and add seasoning as you reheat until steamy. Serve hot

This soup is so delicious that it carries the danger of preventing other parts of the meal being eaten after your family or guests fill up on it.

66. Asparagus and Chicken Noodle Casserole

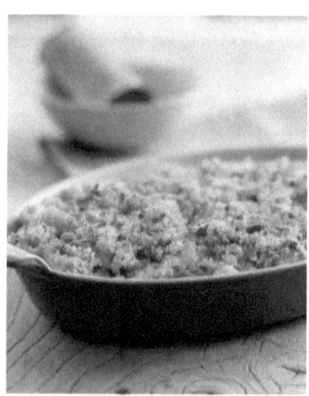

This comforting meal will give you a change from the usual and it is so flavorful that it will turn you into a fan for life.

Ingredients

- 2 bunch trimmed asparagus
- 8 ounces dry and wide noodles of choice
- 2 minced cloves of garlic
- 2 tablespoons each of flour, virgin olive oil and butter
- ½ cup chopped onions

- 1 cup cream of mushroom soup
- 3 cups milk
- Salt and pepper to taste
- Flesh of a whole chicken, cooked and cubed
- 6 ounces grated cheddar cheese
- ½ cup bread crumbs

Method

1. Place the asparagus in a pot of boiled and salted water and cook for a minute. Remove and rinse in cold water then set aside. Use same water to cook noodles following package instructions, less a minute cooking time, drain and stand. Preheat oven to 175 degrees C. Saute onions for 3 minutes over low heat in melted butter. Stir in flour and garlic and cook for a further 2 minutes, stirring.

2. Add in the mushroom soup, milk and seasoning and continue to stir briskly until it thickens. Remove from heat and add to the noodles. Add chicken, half the cheese and asparagus and combine thoroughly. Place mixture into an oven-proof dish and sprinkle the remaining cheese on top. Thoroughly mix together the olive oil and bread crumbs and spread mixture over casserole. Bake for 30 minutes until nicely browned.

Did You Know?

There is a museum in Germany, solely dedicated to asparagus. You get info about its history, how it is cultivated and many other aspects of this vegetable, dubbed 'The food of the gods' by one of the ancient Egyptian queens.

67. Harvest Port and Butternut Squash Stew

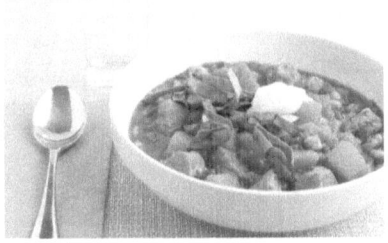

If you want a home cooked meal of restaurant quality, taste and flavor; this is it. You get the best of both worlds in one.

Ingredients

- 3 tablespoons flour
- 1 tablespoon each of olive oil and paprika
- 1 teaspoon each of ground coriander and salt
- pound boneless pork shoulder, cubed
- 2 cups each of chicken broth and peeled and cubed butternut
- 1 cup each of undrained diced tomatoes and thawed frozen corn
- 1 can baby lima beans
- 1 chopped onion
- 2 tablespoons vinegar
- 1 bay leaf

Method

1. Mix thoroughly 2 tablespoons of the flour, coriander, paprika and salt. Thoroughly coat pork and shake off access. Heat oil in a large thick base saucepan and brown the pork a little at a time. Place into crock pot and add all ingredients except flour, beans and broth.

2. Separately combine flour and broth and mix until smooth. Stir into the crock pot and cook covered over low heat for 9 hours. Add the baby lima beans 30 minutes before end of cooking time. Remove from pot and discard bay leaf before serving.

Note

You can substitute the baby lima beans for edamame of frozen cut green beans and the stew would still taste good.

68. Halibut and Corn Chowder

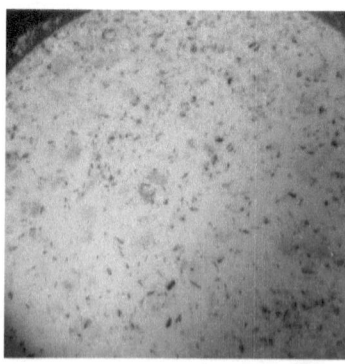

This is a versatile soup you can use with many dishes. You can use any firm fish in place of halibut and you can also experiment with different spices and seasoning.

Ingredients

- 1 red potato, cubed
- ½ large onion, chopped
- ½ cup each of milk and chopped celery
- 1x8 ounces can low sodium chicken broth
- ½ minced garlic clove
- ½ teaspoon salt
- ¼ teaspoon dried marjoram
- 1 tablespoon each of flour and butter
- 1 can each of cream-style corn and drained de-boned and flaked halibut
- 1 cup heavy cream

Method

1. Mix potatoes, celery, onion, garlic, chicken broth, marjoram and salt on a saucepan. Bring to boil over medium heat, reduce heat and simmer for 10 minutes. Whisk in the cream, milk. Mix corn and flour then stir mixture into soup. Heat until slightly thickened, do not allow mixture to boil. Add the fish and stir gently to avoid flaking. Allow to heat through before serving.

Fast tip

This soup is rather pale and leaving the skin on the potatoes will give it a bit of color.

69. Pork Kebabs with Honey

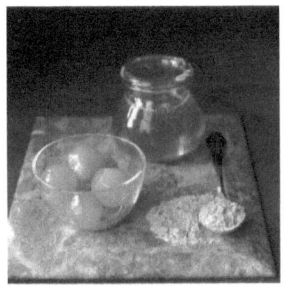

Pork is high in protein, making it filling and able to keep hunger away for longer. The dish therefore offers you comfort without making you feel guilty about it.

Ingredients

- 1½ pounds pork rashers without rind
- 6 peeled and halved baby onions
- 1 tablespoon mustard
- 3 tablespoons honey

Method

1. Preheat oven to 200 °C. Thread the meat onto kebab skewers alternating with the onions. Mix honey and mustard and use mixture to brush kebabs. Arrange on oven rack and bake for 12-15 minutes.

Did you know?

Pope John Paul XXII loved mustard so much that he created a new Vatican position of mustard-maker to the pope in the early 1300s.

70. Four Bean Salad

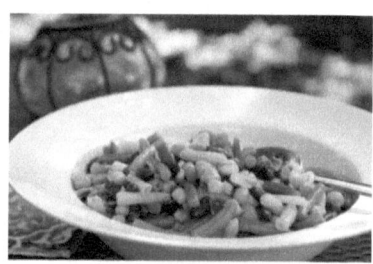

This salad tastes great and is a great source of energy. It will ensure that you do not get hunger pangs every now and again. In addition, beans are very nutritious and are a high-level protein food.

Ingredients

- 1 ½ cups blanched green beans
- 1 cups cooked speckled red beans
- 1 1/4 cups cooked white beans
- 1 each of green peppers medium onions, sliced
- ½ cup each white vinegar and olive oil

- 1 ½ tablespoons caster sugar
- ¼ cup chopped fresh coriander
- Salt and pepper

Method

1. Mix beans, peppers and onions in a salad bowl. Place remaining ingredients into a jug and whisk to make the salad dressing. Drizzle salad dressing over salad and immediately serve.

Olives Fun Fact

The olive tree lives for hundreds of years and olives are harvested for the first time after a tree is 15 years old. Fresh oil tastes better and is better used for salads and after a year it is better used for cooking.

71. Crock Pot Jambalaya

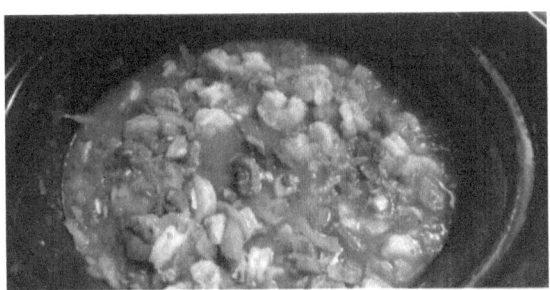

Jambalaya is a favorite in many American households and likely to bring back the memories of the good old days.

Ingredients

- 1 cup chopped onion
- 1 cup chopped green pepper
- 1 cup chopped celery
- 2 garlic cloves, minced
- 1 28 ounces can un-drained diced tomatoes
- ¾ pound cooked prawns
- 2 cups turkey sausage or smoked sausage
- ¼ teaspoon each of hot sauce and pepper
- ½ teaspoon each of salt and dried thyme
- 1 tablespoon dried parsley

Method

1. Add all ingredients except prawns and stir well. Cook on high for 3-4 hours. Add prawns to crock pot for the last 15 minutes of cooking time.

Note

There are variant types of prawns and you can easily substitute one for the other though they may slightly differ in flavor and taste.

72. Sweet Potato Fish Cakes

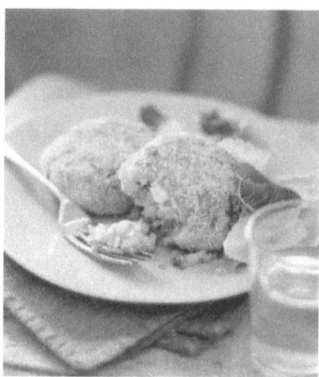

Fish cakes are nutritious and give you the desired comfort and they are a healthy snack that gives you no guilt feelings.

Ingredients

- 1-pound hake or whiting steaks
- 2 sweet potatoes, cooked and mashed
- 1 onion, grated
- 3 tablespoons chopped parsley
- 2 teaspoons lemon juice
- 2 beaten eggs
- 4 tablespoons coconut flour
- Salt and pepper

Method

1. Grease your crock pot. Put fish into blender and blend slightly. Mix fish with rest of ingredients. Shape mixture into six cakes. Sprinkle

flour on a board and roll the fish cakes. Place individually in crock pot. Close and cook on medium for four hours. Put in oven and grill for 2 minutes before serving.

Did you know?

Eggs contain proteins, folic acid and vitamin D. These increase alertness, a lack of vitamin D is associated with depression and reduced mental function.

73. Sweet Potato Fritters

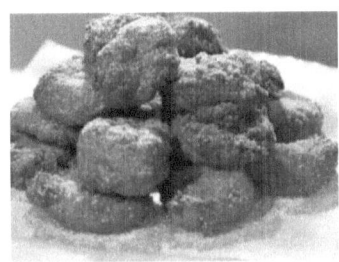

Sweet potato snacks will keep you full for longer and therefore help you eat less and, the sweet variety of potatoes is the healthier cousin.

Ingredients

- 1 pound grated sweet potatoes
- 10 ounces chopped onions
- ½ cup almond flour
- 1 beaten egg
- 1 teaspoon mixed spice
- Salt and pepper
- 2 tablespoon coconut oil

Method

1. Thoroughly mix all ingredients except oil in a bowl. Heat oil in pan and spoon mixture into pan to make several fritters. Slightly press spooned mixture. Fry until crispy and browned then turn and repeat.

Did you know?

Sweet potatoes are versatile vegetables which you can enjoy boiled, fried, roasted, baked, pureed, steamed or grilled.

74. Brown Sugar Barbecue Chicken

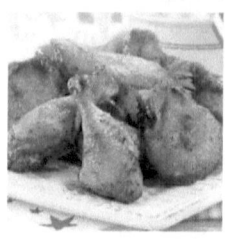

Even the pickiest of eaters are likely to be taken in by this simple and sweet sauce. You will get all the comfort and it really is finger licking good.

Ingredients

- 2 cups tomato sauce
- 1 cup brown sugar
- 2 tablespoons each of Worcestershire sauce and vinegar
- Salt and pepper
- 6 pounds chicken drumettes

Method

1. Preheat oven to 220 degrees C. Whisk together all ingredients except chicken. Use aluminum foil to line 2 baking trays. Toss chicken with one cup sauce then divide them into the two baking trays Bake on top shelves for 35 minutes, turning them after 15 minutes. When done, toss with ½ cup sauce and use remaining sauce for serving.

Did You Know?

Drumettes are the thickest part of a chicken wing, which resembles a small drumstick.

75. Chicken and Sweetcorn Macaroni

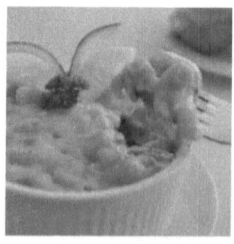

Macaroni and cheese dishes are children's favorites and you can never go wrong with this combination. Add chicken to the duo and you are good to go.

Ingredients

- 2 boiled cups each of macaroni and shredded chicken
- 1 cup each of water and sweetcorn
- 4 ounces butter or margarine
- 2 cups milk
- 3 ounces plain flour
- 1 cup grated cheddar cheese
- ½ teaspoon mustard powder
- Salt and pepper seasoning

Method

1. Preheat oven to 200 degrees C. In a pan over medium heat, melt 1-ounce butter. Add an ounce flour, salt, mustard powder and pepper, mixing thoroughly.

2. Gradually but briskly whisk in the milk and water. Reduce heat and cook while stirring continuously. Remove from heat after sauce thickens. Add macaroni, chicken, ¾ cup cheese and sweetcorn and mix thoroughly. Pour into greased baking dish and top with remainder of cheese. Bake until golden brown then serve hot.

Note

For variety, you can substitute chicken with pork chops but make sure to remove all fat first.

76. Confetti Spaghetti Salad

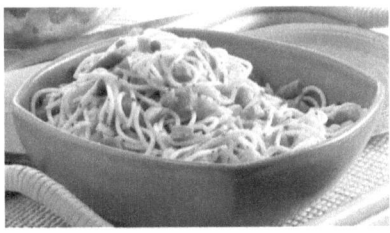

This is an appetizing comfort dish with a colorful appeal. It is very easy to prepare and also has few and easily obtainable ingredients

Ingredients

- 1 7 ounces packet spaghetti, uncooked and broken into thirds
- 2 cups frozen mixed vegetables
- ¼ cup onion, chopped
- ¾ cup chopped tomato
- ½ cup salad dressing

Method

1. Boil spaghetti in a large saucepan with a lot of water and add frozen vegetables in last five minutes. Drain and allow to cool. In a medium sized bowl, toss all ingredients gently and thoroughly mixed. Cover salad and refrigerate for 45 minutes to an hour before serving.

Did you know?

There are more than 600 pasta shapes produced worldwide and most are found in particular regions of the world and not in the others.

77. Beef and Curry Pasta

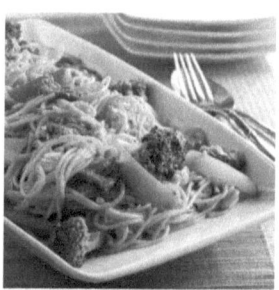

This is an appetizing, scrumptious and filling dish which will keep you going for hours. The curry is just enough to make you feel all fuzzy inside.

Ingredients

- pound macaroni
- 4 teaspoons curry paste
- 1 cup milk
- 3 tablespoons fish sauce
- 2 pounds steak or chuck roast in sizable pieces
- 8 ounces mushrooms
- Medium onion and carrot both sliced thinly

- 10 ounces cauliflower florets
- 2 teaspoons salt
- ½ teaspoon pepper
- 12 ounces trimmed fresh green beans

Method

1. Whisk the paste, milk and sauce in the slow cooker. Add remaining ingredients except beans and stir to ensure sauce coats everything. Add beans but do not mix. Cook on low heat for 8 hours, in the last 30 minutes, stir in beans at ten-minute intervals. Cook pasta according to packet instructions in the last 15 minutes before curry is done. Put drained pasta on a serving dish and top with curry.

Did you know?

Mushrooms are some of the oldest living vegetables and have been used as medicine for thousands of years.

78. Tandoori Chicken

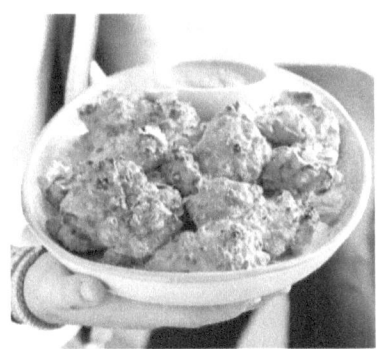

A dish that will make you forget the here and the now as it takes you back to the old days when the stress of adult life fell on someone's shoulders.

Ingredients

- 1 cup, thick and plain yogurt
- 1 garlic clove, crushed
- Peeled and grated ginger piece
- 1 tablespoon each of lemon juice and olive oil
- 1 teaspoon each of masala and ground coriander
- ½ teaspoon each of chili powder and turmeric

- 6 chicken thigh fillets, trimmed
- Cooked rice

Method

1. Mix well yogurt, ginger, garlic, lemon juice, spices, oil and salt in a large bowl. Double slit the top of each thigh without cutting all the way through. Put chicken in mixture making sure to coat well. Refrigerate for 3½ hours.

2. Preheat oven to 220 degrees C towards the end of the refrigeration time. Place chicken in a lined dish and roast until thoroughly cooked. Serve with the rice.

79. Spiced Salmon with Chili Sauce

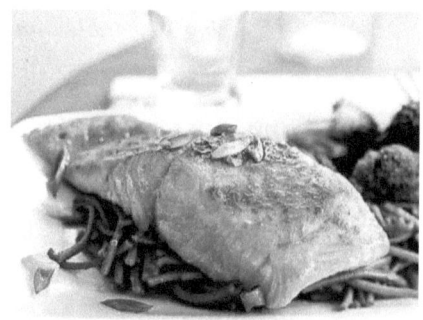

With only 325 calories per serving, this dish is a sure way of enjoying good food while losing weight. The dish gives you comfort without guilt.

Ingredients

- 4 x 6 ounces salmon fillets
- 2 teaspoon chili sauce
- 1 teaspoon honey
- ¼ teaspoon each of ground red pepper, ground turmeric and salt
- ⅛ teaspoon garlic powder

Method

1. Preheat cooking spray coated broiler. Combine all ingredients except the fish in a bowl and stir with a fork. Rub mixture evenly over fish. Place fillets on broiler, skin-side down. Broil for 8-10 minutes.

Did you know?

The spices in this dish will help speed up the metabolic process and therefore help you shed any weight you might want to or help you maintain your weight even as you enjoy comfort food.

80. Slow Cooked Stuffed Gammon

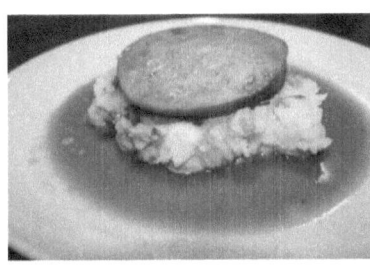

The main ingredient in this dish is beef, and beef is one of the greatest sources of protein. Beef will help you get to the desired amount of proteins per day and because it has no carbs, you can be sure you keep on track of your desired weight loss endeavor.

Ingredients

- 4 pounds boneless gammon
- 1 1 tablespoon oil
- 2 tablespoons curry paste
- 1 cup cooked couscous
- 1 cup dried apples, chopped
- 1 cup dried cranberries
- ½ cup each of pine nuts and maple syrup
- 2 tablespoons vegetable stock
- 2 tablespoon course mustard
- Salt and pepper

Method

1. Grease the crock pot. Make a big hole in the center of the gammon using a flat, sharp knife. Heat oil in a saucepan and add curry, couscous, apples, cranberries and nuts. Season well, remove from the pan and leave to cool.

2. Stuff into gammon and secure with kitchen string. Place in crock pot. Close and cook for 6 hours on low heat. In a bowl, combine syrup,

stock and mustard. Pour over gammon and cook again for two hours. Place in oven to brown.

Did you know?

Berries are good for your memory. They contain flavonoids which can improve memory, learning and general cognitive function including reasoning, decision making and verbal comprehension.

81. Potato and Pork Bake

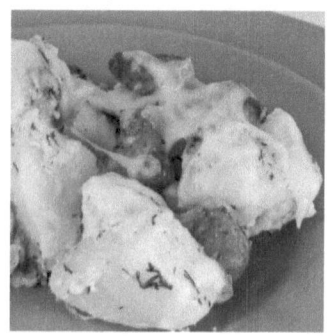

Potatoes are the ultimate comfort food as they always take you back many years. The starchy make up gives the potato its filling quality.

Ingredients

- 8 potatoes cubed
- 8 thick cut pork chops
- 1 onion chopped
- 250 ml vegetable stock

Method

1. Preheat oven to 200 degrees C. Place the potatoes in a baking tray. Arrange the chops over the potatoes. Fry onion until slightly browned and mix with stock. Pour this over the meat and potatoes. Bake for 30 to 40 minutes.

Did You Know?

The now so common vegetable was at some time in its history considered inedible and even poisonous.

82. Summer Cabbage Soup with Sausages

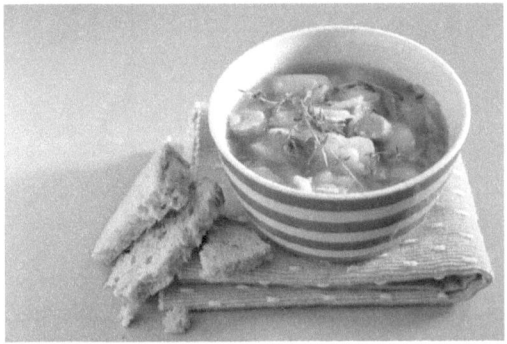

The sausage and cabbage combination in this dish makes the dish highly feeling and ensures loss of weight through keeping you full for longer.

Ingredients

- 4 tablespoons oil
- 1 chopped onion
- 1 sprig thyme
- 8 ounces pork sausages, cooked and sliced
- 1 cabbage, shredded
- 4 medium potatoes, cubed
- 6 cups vegetable stock
- Pepper to taste

Method

1. Heat the oil in a saucepan. Fry the onions in oil until soft. Add the remaining ingredients. Cover and cook for 10-15 minutes. Season well and serve.

Did you know?

Potatoes contain nutrients like vitamin C, B and potassium which are good for relieving inflammation of the intestines and the digestive system.

83. Teriyaki Fried Rice with Chicken

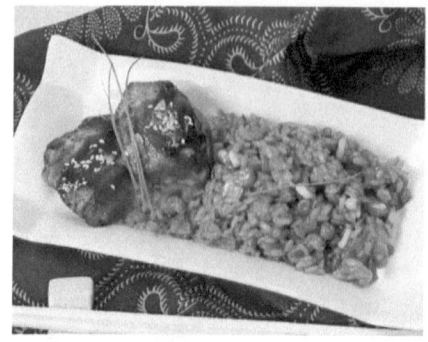

Any meal with chicken is guilt-free comfort food. Chicken is high in protein and therefore low in calories. This allows you to enjoy your food without worrying about weight gain.

Ingredients

- 5 ounces chicken breasts
- 1½ tablespoon vegetable oil
- 2 onions, chopped
- Small carrot, julienned
- Small beaten egg
- 2½ cups cold cooked rice
- 2 tablespoons roasted garlic teriyaki marinade and sauce
- 1 teaspoon chili paste
- 1 tablespoon soy sauce

Method

1. Cut chicken into thin strips. Heat oil in large skillet over high heat. Place chicken, onions, carrot and chili sauce into skillet and stir-fry until chicken is cooked. Gently stir in the egg until firm then add rice and cook until thoroughly heated. Add Teriyaki and soy sauce before you remove from heat and mix well.

Fun fact

Over 50 billion chickens are reared annually for their meat and eggs, making chickens the most populous bird in the world.

84. Sea Bass with Orange and Honey

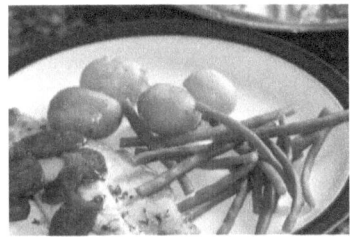

Honey is a naturally warming delicacy whose inclusion here gives the dish a comforting quality that is unmatched.

Ingredients

- 2 large sea-bass fillets
- Zest and juice ½ orange
- 2 teaspoon each honey and mustard
- 2 tablespoon olive oil
- 9 ounces ready-to-eat lentils
- 3 ounces watercress
- Small bunch each parsley and dill, chopped

Method

1. Heat oven to 200^0C. Place fillets skin-down on individual foils. Mix honey, zest, mustard, ½ oil and some seasoning; drizzle mixture over fillets. Pull foil sides up and twist edges. Place foils on baking tray and bake for 10-12 minutes. Warm lentils and mix with remaining ingredients. Divide into 2 plates, place fish on top and drizzle any left juices and serve

85. Slow Cooker Breakfast Casserole

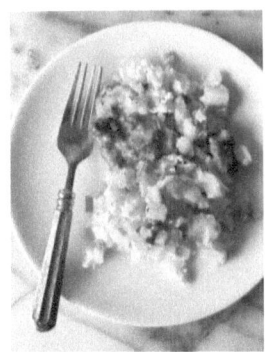

This dish is a filling breakfast dish that has essential nutrients to keep you going and fulfilled for several hours.

Ingredients

- ½ pound ground sausage, browned and drained
- 6 large eggs
- ½ cup milk
- pound frozen hash-browns
- ½ cup salsa
- ½ cup grated cheddar cheese
- ½ pound potatoes
- Salt and pepper to taste

Method

1. Spray non-stick cooking spray into the crock pot. Thoroughly mix together beaten eggs, milk and the salt and pepper before pouring into the cooker. Add the remaining ingredients and stir a little. Cook on low heat for six hours until mixture sets at the center.

Did you know?

Eggs are good for alertness. The protein in egg is an essential component of neurotransmitters like dopamine and norepinephrine which help communication between brain cells.

86. Slow Cooker Jambalaya

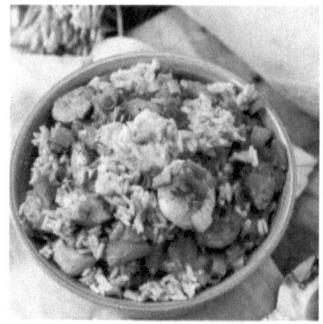

This dish is rich in spices and spices are known for greatly aiding weight loss. Spices are known to speed up metabolism which in turn helps you lose weight faster.

Ingredients

- 1 cup chopped onion
- 1 cup chopped green pepper
- 1 cup chopped celery
- 2 garlic cloves, minced
- 1 28 ounces can un-drained diced tomatoes
- ¾ pound cooked prawns
- 2 cups turkey sausage or smoked sausage
- ¼ teaspoon each of hot sauce and pepper
- ½ teaspoon each of salt and dried thyme
- 1 tablespoon dried parsley

Method

1. Add all ingredients except prawns and stir well. Cook on high for 3-4 hours. Add prawns to crock pot for the last 15 minutes of cooking time.

Did you know?

Tomato is not a vegetable but a fruit and that it helps keep you focused. It also has the potential of positive mood creation and overall clarity.

87. Spaghetti Bolognaise

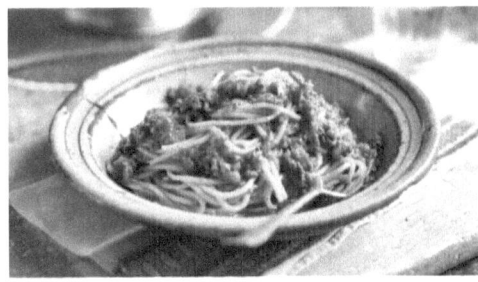

This is a tasty comfort and filling dish which will remind you of those by-gone days and keep you going for hours.

Ingredients

- 1 tablespoon olive oil
- 200 g beef mince
- 1 small onion, sliced

- A chopped garlic clove
- 50 g grated carrots
- 400g tin chopped tomatoes
- 200ml beef stock
- 200 g spaghetti
- Salt and pepper

Method

1. Heat a little oil and fry mince over low heat until browned. Remove from pan and add remaining oil, fry onions until softened. Add garlic and seasoning then fry for two more minutes. Add carrot, mince and tomatoes, stir well to mix.

2. Stir in stock and allow to simmer gently. Cook pasta according to packet instructions. When pasta is cooked, drain and add to sauce and mix well.

Did you know?

In some cultures, garlic is not only considered good for health but even for keeping evil spirits at bay.

88. Beef and Vegetable Parmesan

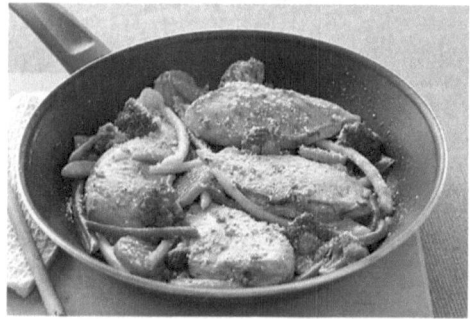

This tasty comfort dish has easily available ingredients has a total of only between 2225 and 2300kj per serving. It has net carbs of 7g per serving.

Ingredients

- pound boneless beef sirloin
- 4 cups broccoli florets
- 2 cups cauliflower florets

- 5 tablespoons shredded parmesan cheese
- 2-3 tablespoons olive oil
- Salt and freshly ground pepper

Method

1. Cut beef into sizable pieces. Sprinkle seasoning. Put a layer of the vegetables on the crock pot. Place the meat on top and add the remaining vegetables on the sides and on top of the meat. Add about 50 milliliters of water. Cook on medium heat for 3-4 hours. Sprinkle the cheese on top before serving.

Did you know?

Olive oil is rich in the anti-oxidant hydroxytyrosol. Anti-oxidants help protect the body against the damage caused by free radicals. The fresher the olive oil, the better the taste and the flavor.

89. Fried Green Tomatoes

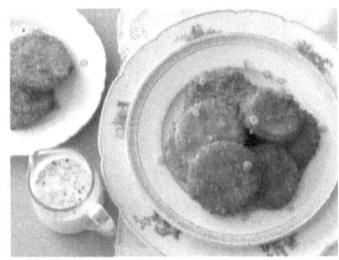

Comfort eating with an easy cooking method and few ingredients is difficult to resist and this is one such a dish with the additional pleasure of great taste.

Ingredients

- 1 lightly beaten egg
- ½ cup each of cornmeal mix, flour and buttermilk
- Salt and pepper
- 2 large green tomatoes sliced 5mm thick
- 1 cup vegetable oil

Method

1. Whisk buttermilk and egg. Mix together cornmeal, ½ the flour and salt and pepper in a mixing bowl. Coat tomatoes in remaining flour

before dipping into egg and buttermilk mixture then coat with cornmeal mixture.

2. Heat oil in skillet over high heat and reduce heat when oil begins smoking. Gently place coated tomatoes in batches and cook until golden. Remove from oil and drain. Season before serving.

Note

Buttermilk is called for in many recipes even though it is not as widely used as it used to be. You can therefore use substitutes for the milk and this won't change the taste if you use a substitute with an acid to maintain the characteristic flavor.

90. Mushroom and Cabbage Stroganoff

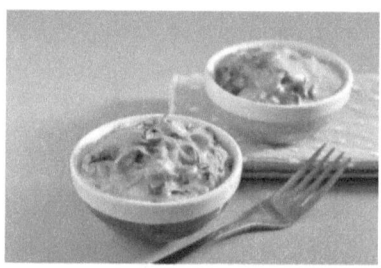

It is not every time that you get comfort food that has the potential to aid in weight loss. The protein in this dish is obtained from the mushrooms and keeps you full for a long time and prevents hunger pangs.

Ingredients

- 4 tablespoons oil
- 1 large onion, chopped
- 2 tablespoons paprika
- 4 pounds sliced mushrooms
- 1 white and 1 red cabbages, shredded
- 3½ cups vegetable stock
- pound double cream
- Salt and pepper

Method

1. Heat oil in a large frying pan. Add onions and fry until soft. Add paprika, cabbage and mushrooms and cook for 3 minutes. Add stock

and simmer covered, for 8 minutes. Add the cream and season well then cook for a further 4 minutes before serving

Did you know?

Cabbage is a cruciferous vegetable a type of vegetables linked to significant reduction in risk of variant cancers. In addition, cabbage can stop running tummies and improve appetite.

91. Beef and Portobello Stroganoff

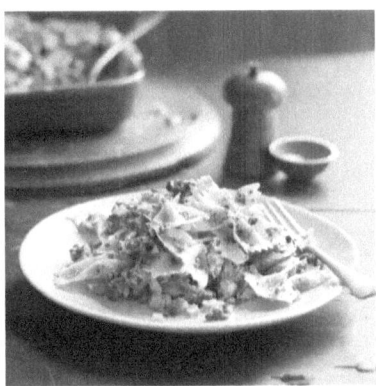

Comfort food with many health benefits from nutrient rich mushrooms. Most mushroom types are even good for your bladder because of the presence of the mineral selenium.

Ingredients

- 4 tablespoons oil
- 1 large onion, chopped
- 2 tablespoons paprika
- 4 pounds sliced Portobello mushrooms
- 2 pounds cubed beef
- 3½ cups vegetable stock
- 1-pound double cream
- Salt and pepper

Method

1. Heat oil in a large frying pan and fry beef until tender and browned. Add onions and fry until soft. Add paprika and mushrooms and cook for 5 minutes. Add stock and simmer covered, for 12 minutes. Add

the cream and season well then cook for a further 6 minutes before serving.

Note

There are poisonous varieties of mushrooms and most mushrooms are also easily affected by the surrounding plants and trees so be careful about the mushrooms if they are not store bought.

92. Chili Con Carne

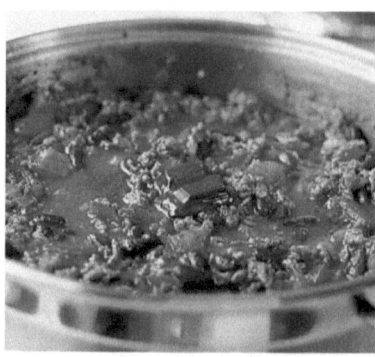

This dish gives you a lot of freedom to maneuver as you can include and drop off some ingredients which are not main, and still come out with a good dish.

Ingredients

- Pound minced beef
- 1 medium sized onion, chopped
- 3 finely chopped garlic cloves
- ½ tablespoon each of ground cumin and dried oregano
- 1 tablespoon ground chili peppers
- Salt and pepper seasoning
- 1 cup each of beef broth, cooked kidney beans and tomato puree
- 1 large tomato, chopped
- Cheddar cheese, grated
- Chopped onion

Method

1. Sauté ground beef, onion and garlic in a saucepan until meat changes color. Drain off and discard fat. Add all ingredients except beans then allow to simmer for 3-4 hours, pot uncovered. In last 30 minutes of

cooking, add beans, mix thoroughly and continue to simmer. Taste and adjust seasoning if desired.

Did You Know?

You would enjoy the chili better if you allow the flavors to mingle overnight, refrigerated. So, if possible, prepare dish a day before then reheat when you are ready to serve.

93. Baked Sweet Potatoes with Sour Cream

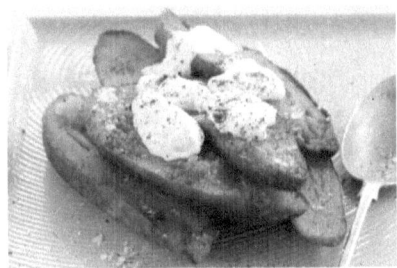

This is a fairly easy dish to make and you can have it ready in just over an hour both prep and cooking time.

Serves: 2

Ingredients

- 2 medium sized sweet potatoes, scrubbed
- ¼ cup sour cream
- ½ tablespoon maple syrup

Method

1. Preheat oven to 220 degrees C. Pierce potatoes with a fork and bake on lined baking tray for 50 minutes. Remove from oven and slit potatoes open making sure not to reach the opposite side. Push ends to create an opening. Mix sour cream and maple syrup in a bowl and put a portion in the potato opening. Serve.

Note

Potatoes contain Vitamin C and Vitamin B6. With 132calories for every 100g potato, they are diet friendly and appetite satisfying at the same time.

94. Breakfast Barley with Sunflower Seeds and Banana

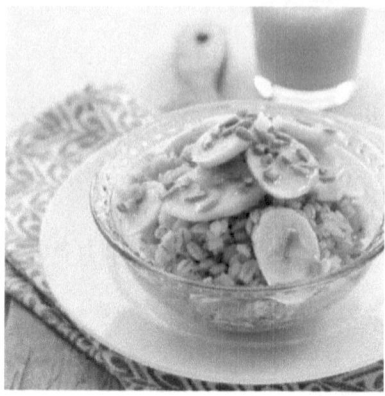

If you are tired of oatmeal and looking for a hale and hearty start to your day, you can swap with this crispy breakfast bowl. The combination of banana and barley provides almost eight grams of resistant starch and metabolism-boosting fiber that makes this dish an ultra-satisfying morning meal. A sprinkling of sunflower seeds and a spoonful of honey give this energetic dish a delicious sweet-and-salty finish.

Ingredients

- 1 teaspoon honey
- 1 tablespoon unsalted sunflower seeds
- 1 sliced banana
- 1/3 cup of raw quick-cooking pearl barley
- 2/3 cup water

Method

1. Add barley and 2/3 cup of water in a small microwave-safe bowl. Keep the microwave on at HIGH for six minutes. Blend it for two minutes. Top with honey, sunflower seeds and banana slices.

Facts to know

Barley has its hunger-fighting reputation and after having barley in breakfast, blood sugar can be on an even level for a longer period of time. This is for the reason that the carbs in barley are "low glycemic index," and they raise blood sugar little by little than some other carbohydrate foods. This can help to make you feel less hungry.

95. Curried Egg Salad Sandwich

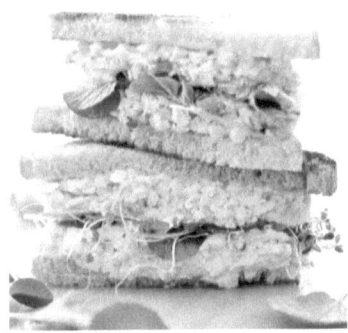

This egg salad recipe can be a healthy new way to bring about eggs into lunchtime. The use of low-fat Greek yogurt instead of mayo cut back the calories and fat alongside the curry powder provides a shake of antioxidants. If you want to save preparation time, you can batch-cook a dozen of eggs at the starting of each week.

Ingredients

- Two hard-cooked and chopped eggs
- One orange
- Two slices rye bread, toasted
- 1/8 teaspoon pepper
- 1/8 teaspoon salt
- 1/4 teaspoon curry powder
- Two tablespoons chopped red bell pepper
- 1/2 cup of fresh spinach
- Two tablespoons pure Greek-style low-fat yogurt

Method

1. Take eggs, pepper, salt, curry powder, bell pepper, and yogurt in a small bowl; mix these well. Put spinach on rye bread, top with egg salad, and serve up the dish with pieces of orange on the side.

Facts to know

Eggs are just the perfect food for dieters. They're low in calories (only eighty calories per egg), tasty and filled with fulfilling protein that helps curb cravings.

96. Salmon Noodle Bowl

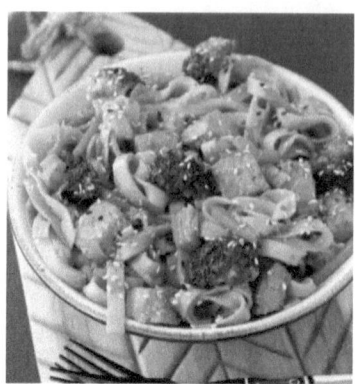

This thirty-minute meal provides a gift of metabolism-boosting and nutritious ingredients in a single bowl. The avocado and salmon are full of hale and hearty fats, and noodles are rich in fiber.

Ingredients

- 1/2 small avocado, shaped into bite-size pieces
- Four ounces cucumber with skin, cut into medium pieces
- 1/4 teaspoon fresh pepper
- 1/4 teaspoon kosher salt
- Three TBSP lime juice
- One tablespoon toasted sesame oil
- One (6-oz) salmon fillet, cut into 8 pieces skin off
- Cooking spray
- Five ounces asparagus, cut in thirds
- Four ounces of soba buckwheat noodles or whole-wheat spaghetti

Method

1. Until getting soft, cook the noodles in boiling water (around eight minutes for spaghetti and six minutes for soba). Put asparagus into the same boiling water and cook about two minutes; finally, clean with cold water.

2. Heat a skillet or grill pan over medium to high heat. With cooking spray coat the pan lightly. Roast the salmon until cooked through. Prepare the vinaigrette: fluff up pepper, salt, lime juice and sesame oil together in a small bowl. Mix the asparagus, noodles, and vinaigrette in a medium sized serving bowl. Add the avocado and cucumber;

blend to coat and add salmon just before serving. Serve the dish hot or at room temperature.

Facts to know

The asparagus used in this dish are the unsung hero, offering a wide range of necessary vitamins and minerals, including iron, folate and vitamins A and C. Omega-3s in salmon assists to build more muscle and more muscle indicate more calories burned.

97. Chicken Chilaquiles and Black Bean

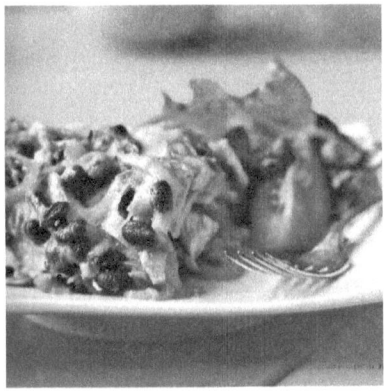

This conventional Mexican breakfast food needs only eight ingredients, including corn tortillas, queso blanco and chicken but per serving it comes in only 2 grams of saturated fat and under 300 calories.

Baking this Mexican dish drops off fat but keeps the savor. Though the conventional Mexican breakfast needs only eight ingredients and you can take it at any time of day; however, you can also mix some brown rice with the beans to get a source of complete protein and can serve with a mixed green salad topped with olives, tomato wedges, and diced avocado.

Ingredients

- 1 cup shredded queso blanco (4 ounces)
- 15 (6-inch) corn tortillas, cut into 1-inch strips
- 1 can salsa de chile fresco (for instance, El Pato)
- 1 cup fat-free, less-sodium chicken broth
- 1 can black beans (15-ounce), drained and rinsed
- 2 cups shredded cooked chicken breast
- 5 garlic cloves, minced

- 1 cup of thinly sliced onion
- Cooking spray

Method

1. Heat a big nonstick skillet over medium to high heat then coat the pan with cooking spray. Put onion there and fry up for five minutes or until they get lightly browned. Add garlic and then cook it for one minute. Next, add chicken and cook it for thirty seconds. Move this mixture to a medium bowl; mix beans with it. Add salsa and broth to the pan; lessen the heat and cook for five minutes. Finally, put it to one side.

2. Put half of tortilla strips in a baking dish coated with cooking spray. Place half of chicken mixture over tortillas; pour the remaining chicken mixture and tortillas over it. Pour broth mixture uniformly over the chicken and tortillas mixture. Add cheese. After that bake it at 450° for ten minutes or until the cheese is melted and tortillas get lightly browned.

Facts to know

Black beans in this dish are filled with fiber and high protein that make them another weight-loss super food.

98. Pan-grilled Salmon with Pineapple Salsa

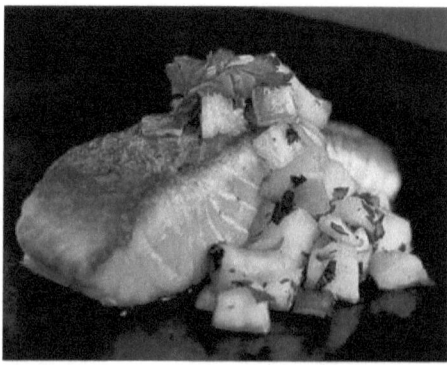

To get a successful weight loss plan, lean protein is an indispensable ingredient. And salmon is that source of lean protein which is not only best in quality but also has the added advantage of being filled with monounsaturated fats.

These healthy fats have been proven as a natural support to weight loss. This can be a wonderful dish for a summer night. You can also add fiber with it with half a cup of whole-grain rice.

Ingredients

- 4 (6-ounce) salmon fillets (about 1/2-inch thick)
- 1/8 teaspoon ground red pepper
- 1/2 teaspoon salt
- Cooking spray
- 1 tablespoon rice vinegar
- 2 tablespoons chopped cilantro
- 2 tablespoons finely chopped red onion
- 1 cup chopped fresh pineapple

Method

1. Take chopped pineapple, chopped cilantro, onion, rice vinegar and red pepper in a bowl; put the bowl to one side. Heat a nonstick grill pan over a medium to high heat and coat with cooking spray. Add salt and fish. Cook the fish for nearly four minutes on each side or until it comes off easily when tested with a fork. Finally serve the dish topping with salsa.

Facts to know

Fish is a prominent source of lean protein. And on the whole salmon is superior as it contains bounty of heart-healthy fats called omega 3s.

99. Italian Garbanzo Salad

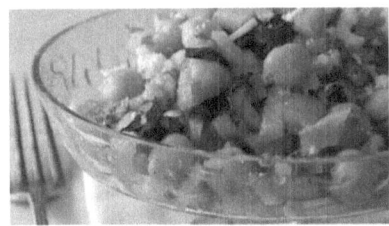

This vegan salad is a classic example of the Mediterranean diet which is well-known for its knack to support overall health. You can take this salad as a first course of a meal or as a side to grilled chicken. This recipe is meatless, low cholesterol and gluten-free.

Ingredients

- 2 cans of chickpeas (garbanzo beans), drained and rinsed
- 3 cups of finely chopped fennel bulb
- 1/2 cup of (2 ounces) crumbled feta cheese
- 1/4 teaspoon salt
- 1 tablespoon olive oil
- 1/3 cup of balsamic vinegar
- 1 cup of chopped fresh basil
- One 3/4 cups finely chopped red onion
- 2 cups of chopped tomato
- 4 garlic cloves, minced
- 1 teaspoon freshly ground black pepper

Method

1. Except the cheese, mix all ingredients in a bowl; toss it well. Keep it for thirty minutes; Finally, add the cheese.

Facts to know

Garbanzo beans (chickpeas) are a huge source of fiber and soy protein. Over all, this salad attributes a number of the diet's key pillars: lean protein (chickpeas), healthy fats (olive oil), fresh vegetables (onion, tomato), low-fat dairy (feta cheese), and the nicest thing is per serving (1 cup) the dish is only 160 calories!

100. Greek Yogurt Fruit Parfait

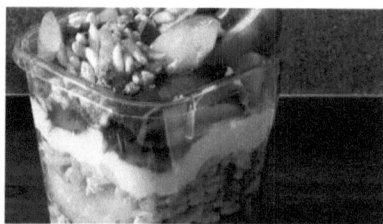

If you're wishing to drop your weight quickly, this parfait can be an awesome breakfast option for you. Each of the ingredients in this recipe endows with a healthy dose of protein and slimming fiber.

This five-minute dish is filling enough for lunch. The creamer and thicker Greek yogurt is more satisfying than regular low-fat yogurt.

Ingredients

- One tablespoon honey, agave nectar or maple syrup
- One tablespoon ground flaxseed
- Two tablespoons almonds and walnuts, chopped and toasted
- 3/4 cup puffed rice cereal
- Two cups sliced mixed plums, nectarines and peaches
- 3/4 cup fat-free plain Greek yogurt

Method

1. In a tall 4-cup jar or container, pour half of the yogurt, syrup, nuts, flaxseed, cereal and fruit. Do it again with the remaining half of ingredients, finishing with syrup (If you wish to have a crunchy parfait, separately add the cereal right before eating). Chill it up to 5 hours.

Facts to know

Researchers have found that people who took a moderate-fat diet including almonds were able to drop more weight than a control group that didn't take nuts. Nuts can aid you to keep your hunger away and promote your metabolism.

101. Toasted Hazelnut, Raw Kale and Grapefruit Salad

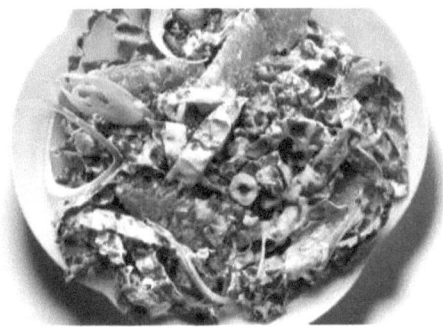

Grapefruit—the scene-stealer of this salad—has a very old standing for driving weight loss. If truth be told, having it at every meal was the source of a fad diet that set out in the 1930s and has made something of a comeback recently.

It is now proven with the recent researches that obese people who take half a grapefruit at the starting of each meal loss more weight than those who don't.

Ingredients

- One ounce (1/3 cup) of chopped and toasted hazelnuts
- Eight ounces of very thinly sliced lacinato kale or baby kale leaves
- 1/4 teaspoon black pepper
- 1/2 teaspoon kosher salt
- Two tablespoons extra-virgin olive oil
- 1/2 cup of fat-free plain yogurt
- 1/4 cup of fresh lemon juice
- 1/2 small red onion, thinly sliced
- Pink grapefruit

Method

1. Slice one/two grapefruit; Chop up 2 rings of onion. Take a large plate and put the chopped onion there with grapefruit juice, pepper, salt, oil, yogurt, and lemon juice. Shake it well until finely mixed. Put the kale into the mix. Top with remaining hazelnuts, grapefruit and onion.

Facts to know

Kale in this salad contains vitamins A, C and K. and grapefruit facilitates the rapidity of weight loss by lowers cholesterol and curbing hunger.

102. Creamy Avocado Cups

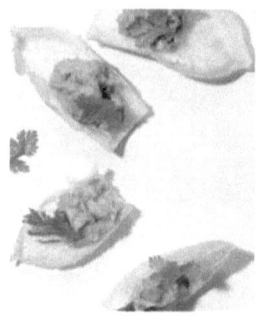

This simple snack will hold back those mid-afternoon hunger cramps with only 30 calories per serving.

Ingredients

- 12 endive leaves
- 1 tablespoon chopped fresh cilantro

- 1/4 teaspoon ground cumin
- 1 tablespoon plain yogurt or reduced-fat sour cream
- 1 tablespoon lime juice
- 1 avocado

Method

1. Pit, peel, and mash one avocado; put it to one side. In another small bowl take plain yogurt or reduced-fat sour cream, chopped fresh cilantro, ground cumin and lime juice; mix the avocado with this. Spoon over the mixture with endive leaves.

Facts to know

The source of this bite's hunger-suppressing power is oleic acid, a fusion found in avocados' natural monounsaturated fats. This acid generates the production of an additional compound in the intestine which fires fullness signals to the brain.

103. Oat Clusters & Dark Chocolate

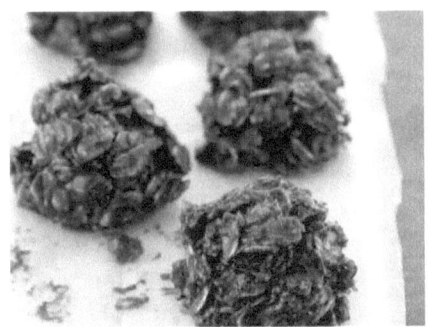

Yes, it is proved that healthy desserts can assist burn fat. This delicious dessert in this recipe provides two appetite-suppressing ingredients: the dark chocolate which is full of healthy fats to facilitate curb cravings and oatmeal which is full of resistant starch.

Ingredients

- 3/4 cup of old-fashioned rolled oats
- 1/4 cup of semisweet chocolate chunks
- Two tablespoons of 1% low-fat milk
- Two tablespoons of peanut butter

Method

1. Heat chocolate chunks, milk, and peanut butter in a saucepan over low heat for three minutes or until the chunks get melt. Whisk oats and remove the pan from heat. Add melon baller or small ice cream scoop with a spoon and keep it in the fridge for ten minutes.

Facts to know

Peanut butter provides the filling protein as well as acts as glue that unites the clusters together and the eventual result of this recipe is the ultimate guilt-free and satisfying treat.

104. Spiced Green Tea Smoothie

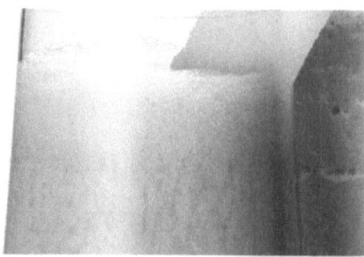

This rich smoothie is just the thing if you get fed up of drinking hot green tea. Savored with agave nectar, cayenne spices and lemon, it offers all the dietary advantages of green tea and will make you rejuvenated. This recipe has low saturated fat, low cholesterol, low calorie and low in sodium.

Ingredients

- 1/8 teaspoon cayenne pepper
- 3/4 cup strong green tea, chilled
- Six to eight ice cubes
- Two tablespoons fat-free plain yogurt
- One small pear, skin on, cut into pieces
- Two teaspoons agave nectar
- Juice of one lemon (2-3 tbsp)

Method

1. After mixing all ingredients together in a blender, blend until it gets smooth. Drink it cold.

Facts to know

Green tea is one of the best fat-burning drink consists of a metabolism-boosting compound known as EGCG. Study has found that drinking four cups of green tea in a day for eight weeks helped people to drop more than six pounds. An antioxidant known as Catech and Caffeine can stimulate nervous system and boost fat-burning thus can facilitate dropping your extra pounds and trim your waist.

105. Chocolate-Dipped Banana Bites

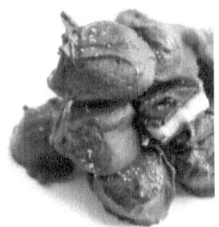

Dessert can also be a healthy meal and help to boost metabolism. You just need a knife and microwave to prepare this easier-than-pie dessert. The bananas in this recipe are a loaded source of resistant starch/healthy carbohydrate which will help you eat less and burn calories. Furthermore, the semisweet chocolate includes healthy fats to promote enhancing your metabolism.

Ingredients

- 1 small banana, peeled and cut into 1-inch chunks
- 2 tablespoons semisweet chocolate chunks

Method

1. Put chocolate chunks in a small microwave-safe bowl or heavy-duty zip-top plastic bag and then melt the chocolate. Pour the liquid chocolate onto the sliced bananas.

Facts to know

Bananas are the loaded source of Resistant Starch and chocolate is an excellent source of metabolism-boosting MUFAs and together you can have a dessert that is a weight-loss winner.

106. Banana & Almond Butter Toast

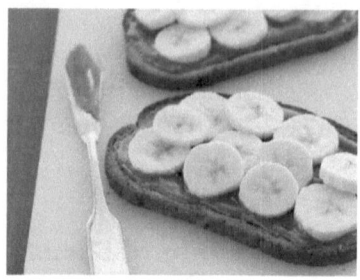

One slice includes less than 300 hundred calories, but it can assure to keep you full until lunchtime. At the same time banana and the rye bread will get you halfway to your daily Resistant Starch goal.

Ingredients

- 1 banana, sliced
- 1 slice rye bread, toasted
- 1 tablespoon almond butter

Method

1. Spurt the almond butter over the toast. Top with banana slices.

Facts to know

This yummy but simple morning pick-me-up offers at least three of the best foods to take for breakfast. The whole-grain rye bread and bananas are high in resistant starch that helps boost up metabolism while the almond butter complements healthy monounsaturated fats and hunger-curbing protein.

107. Honey Grapefruit with Banana

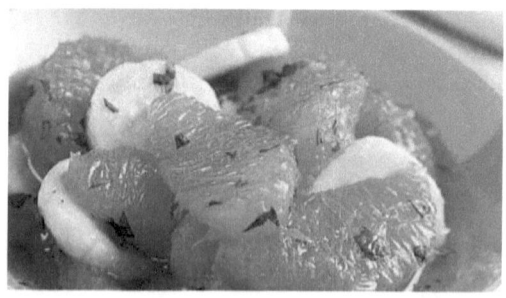

Are you trying to stay slim or trim down? If so, you can't go wrong with this flavorful tropical fruit salad which can be just the right meal for breakfast or as a colorful side dish at lunch. You don't have to throw away sweets on the way to drop your pounds! Fruit could be an excellent substitute to more fattening sweet treats, and it endows with vitamin C and fiber. This Recipe is low sodium, low saturated fat, low fat, low cholesterol, low calorie, gluten-free and diabetic.

Ingredients

- 1 tablespoon honey
- 1 tablespoon fresh chopped mint
- 1 cup sliced banana (about 1)
- About 2 cups (24-ounce) chilled red grapefruit slices

Method

1. Make 1/4 cup of grape juice and reserve the rest grapefruit slices. Mix the juice, grapefruit slices and remaining ingredients in a medium bowl. Toss the mixer gently for a smooth finish. Serve right away, or chill to have it later.

Facts to know

Grapefruit is considered as one of the most effective weight loss foods as it has a considerable effect on insulin, a fat-storage hormone. In addition, it comes up with one of the highest water concentrations of most fruits (nearly 90% of its weight is water), that's why it can fill you up fast and help you avoid overeating.

108. Broccoli and Feta Omelet with Toast

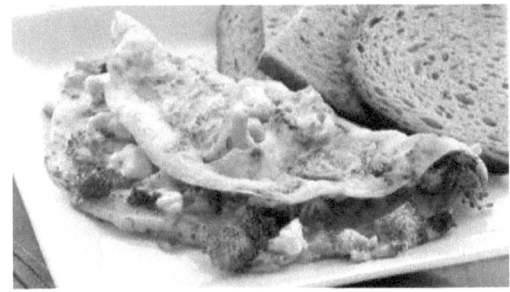

This simple breakfast recipe will make you feel satisfied yet energized and takes only fifteen minutes from start to finish. The protein-loaded eggs and the broccoli which is filled with filling fiber curb your appetite and will help you to hold back those late-morning hunger. You can use either fresh or frozen broccoli for this dish. The feta cheese adds a nice flavor and some CLAs too.

Ingredients

- 2 slices rye bread, toasted
- 1 cup chopped broccoli
- 1/4 teaspoon dried dill
- 2 tablespoons crumbled feta cheese
- 2 large eggs, beaten
- Cooking spray

Method

1. Firstly, heat a nonstick skillet with a medium heat and coat the pan with cooking spray. After that put in broccoli there and cook for 3 minutes. Mix feta cheese, egg and dill in a small bowl. Pour this mixture in to pan and cook it for 3 to 4 minutes; Toss the omelet and fry it as you like. Finally serve this with toast.

Facts to know

Broccoli is that cruciferous veggie that offers you multiple benefits. It is rich in filling fibers, well-known to prevent weight problems and also distinguished for its cancer-preventing power.

109. White Bean & Herb Hummus with Crudites

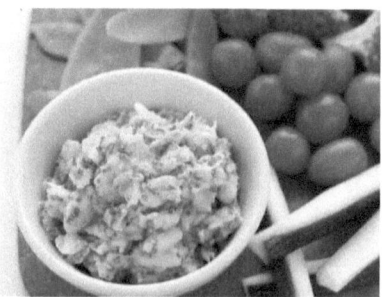

If you are tired of tasteless supermarket hummus, you can try this recipe to whip up a batch of this fiber-rich and savory version in your own kitchen which takes only takes five minutes to prepare. All you need is four ingredients: chives, hearty-healthy olive oil, lemon and—last but not the least—white beans, which have almost 4 grams of resistant starch per serving.

Ingredients

- Various raw vegetables, such as baby carrots, chopped broccoli florets, and sliced red or green peppers
- 2 teaspoons olive oil
- 1 tablespoon lemon juice
- 1 tablespoon chopped chives
- 1/4 cup canned white beans, drained and rinsed

Method

1. Mix oil, lemon juice, beans, and chives in a small bowl. Squash with a fork until it gets smooth. Serve with 1/2 cup of raw vegetables, for instance, broccoli, bell peppers, sugar snap peas, carrots, cucumbers and grape tomatoes.

Facts to know

Beans are economical, versatile, filling and a great source of protein. These are also rich in fiber and dawdling to digest. That indicates you will feel full longer and stay away from eating more.

110. BBQ Turkey Burgers

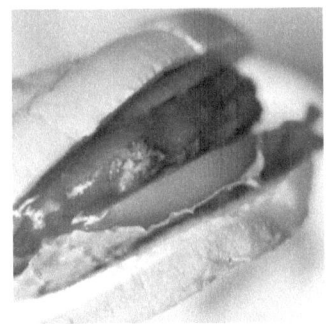

BBQ Turkey Burgers are yummy and ultra- mushy that make them an excellent alternative to conventional high-fat beef patties. Sweet onion in this recipe can also offer you a delicious taste compare to spicy BBQ sauce. You can also try it with grilled pineapple.

Ingredients

- 4 (1.6-oz) toasted sesame seed buns
- pound ground dark-meat turkey

- 1/4 cup barbecue sauce
- 4 slices sweet onion, grilled
- 1/4 teaspoon freshly ground black pepper
- Pinch of kosher salt
- 1/2 teaspoon paprika
- 1/4 teaspoon ground cumin
- 1 garlic clove, minced

Method

1. Gently mix cumin, paprika, garlic and turkey together in medium bowl. Shape the turkey into four 4-inch patties; spice up with pepper and salt. Heat up the grill from medium to high; keep on turning the grill until cooked through (it might take nearly seven minutes per side). Serve with favored buns and toppings.

Facts to know

Lean protein helps you stay fuller for longer and the amino acids in this protein are the building blocks for muscle. These fresh Turkey burgers are an excellent source of lean protein and a wonderful resource of weight-loss food.

111. Middle Eastern Rice Salad

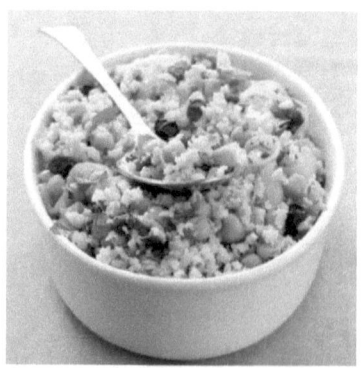

This twenty-minute dish works well equally as a stand-alone or a side meal and is crammed to the brim with healthy ingredients. And when it comes to fat burning, they all do better than the chickpeas.

Simply one half-cup of hearty beans—a staple of Middle Eastern and Mediterranean cuisine— are filled with enough fiber and protein to fill you up without weighing you down.

Ingredients

- 1/4 cup chopped fresh parsley
- 1/4 cup chopped fresh mint
- 1/2 cup chopped pitted dates
- Three cups cooked brown rice
- Freshly ground black pepper
- 1/4 teaspoon salt
- 1/2 teaspoon ground cumin
- Two tablespoons olive oil
- One (16-ounce) can drained and rinsed chickpeas
- About 3/4 cup thinly sliced sweet onion or 1/2 Vidalia.

Method

1. Heat oil in a Take a large nonstick skillet; pour oil in it and heat it over medium to high heat. Put the sliced onion and cook it until the onions start to brown. Take away the skillet from heat, and add salt, cumin and chickpeas. Spice the mix with freshly crushed black pepper.

2. In a large bowl take parsley, mint, dates, onion-chickpea mixture and rice together. Toss thoroughly until it gets mix well. Serve the dish hot or at room temperature.

Facts to know

The chickpeas and the brown rice in this recipe fill more than 4 grams of RS per serving and the dates provide ample of appetite-suppressing fiber which will help you stay full longer.

112. Energy-stimulating Quinoa

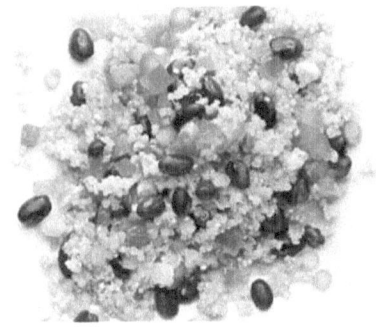

This energy-stimulating Quinoa keeps you stimulated after a workout or between meals. Fragrant spices, fresh veggies and black beans which is another excellent source of fiber complete this satisfying dish. You can take it as a main meal for lunch or as a supplement dish with dinner.

Ingredients

- Splash of freshly ground black pepper
- Drop of salt
- One teaspoon fresh lemon juice
- One teaspoon olive oil
- One sliced scallion
- One cup cooked quinoa
- One small tomato, chopped
- 1/3 cup canned low-sodium black beans, cleaned and drained

Method

1. Take all the ingredients in a medium sized bowl and softly toss to mix it up well.

Facts to know

Quinoa is one of the cool foods around that is filled with fiber and protein and a wonderful combination for those who are looking to keep their metabolism humming and stay energized.

113. Avocado Whip

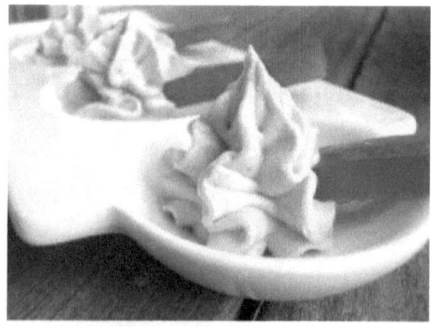

If you are bored with guacamole, you can try creamier alternative, which takes only five minutes to prepare and gets its unique flavor from tahini.

Serve it as a spread on sandwiches or use it as a dip for veggies. Either way, you'll get a lot of heart-healthy monounsaturated fats to accelerate metabolism and keep you feeling full.

Ingredients

- 1/4 teaspoon fresh pepper
- 1/4 teaspoon kosher salt
- 1/4 cup chopped onion
- One tablespoon tahini
- 1/4 cup of fresh lime juice
- Two avocados, peeled and pitted

Method

1. Mix all ingredients in a food processor; process it about 30 seconds or until getting smooth. Take it to a serving dish; cover with plastic wrap and then refrigerate. Decorate with fresh pepper. Finally, serve with one TBSP of lime juice

Facts to know

Because of its combo of essential fatty acids, Avocado can speed up your metabolic rate and the antioxidants help to reduce inflammation.

114. Crisp Chickpea Slaw

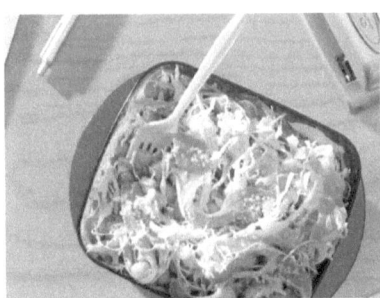

Prepare this slaw for your weekend picnic or weekday lunch. As the cabbage releases moisture that's why you need only a little dressing for the slaw.

Ingredients

- Two tablespoons sesame toasted seeds
- Two carrots, thinly sliced or peeled with a vegetable peeler into strips or 2 cups of frayed carrots

- Two stalks celery, thinly sliced
- Two 1/2 cups of sliced packed green cabbage
- One (15-oz) can of low-sodium chickpeas, cleaned and drained
- Freshly ground black pepper
- One tablespoon water
- One tablespoon cider vinegar
- 1/4 teaspoon kosher salt
- 1/4 cup fat-free plain yogurt

Method

1. Take a medium bowl and mix the pepper, salt, water, vinegar and yogurt. Add the carrots, celery, cabbage and chickpeas; toss to mix well. Spray with sesame seeds. Transfer the slaw to two portable containers or a plastic food-storage bag. Refrigerate it at least four hours before serving; you can keep it up to 3 days.

Facts to know

Garbanzo beans also known as chickpeas are laden with slimming resistant starch. They're also a huge source of fiber and protein which will keep you packed until dinnertime.

115. Spicy Southwestern Black Bean Chili

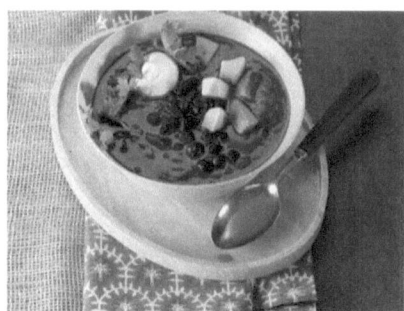

This hearty soup which, per serving, delivers 13 grams of fiber and 17 grams of protein is a yummy preparation that can boost your metabolism hugely.

Ingredients

- 1/4 cup chopped fresh cilantro
- 1/4 cup reduced-fat sour cream
- Two (15.5 ounce) cans black beans, cleaned and drained

- Four (32 ounces) boxes of tomato soup and roasted red pepper and 1 teaspoon ground cumin
- Two tablespoons chili powder
- One finely chopped large garlic clove
- One cup jalapeno, chopped and seeded
- One large chopped onion (about one and half cups)
- Two teaspoons olive oil
- 1/2 cup of firm-ripe diced peeled avocado Cilantro sprigs (optional)

Method

1. Heat the oil in a large saucepan over a medium to high heat; add the jalapeño and onion; stirring and cook until getting softened (about three minutes).

2. Put the cumin, chili powder and garlic; cook for one minute. Mix the black beans and tomato soup; Again, cook for five minutes. Add the chopped cilantro. Pour the soup into bowls; Top with cilantro sprigs, avocado and one tablespoon of sour cream.

Facts to know

This recipe attributes two kinds of hot pepper: jalapeños and chili powder. These peppers with any kind of foods lights a fire under your metabolism and enhance your calorie burn rate.

116. Avocado Peach Salad

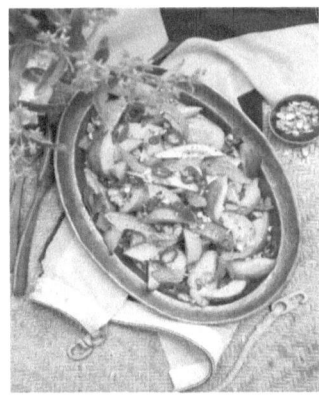

This juicy salad is packed with nutrients and minerals, it is made with peaches, mangoes and tomatoes.

Ingredients

- Any variety greens from your box such as romaine, kale, or Swiss chard.
- 3-5 Peaches Depending on Size
- 1/3-1/2 of an Avocado Depending on the Size of the Salad
- Cherry Tomatoes or Beefsteak Tomatoes
- Oranges
- Herb of Choice like Basil, Italian Parsley, or Cilantro
- Mango
- Bell Peppers

Method

1. Toss in all the ingredients. Enjoy!

Swiss chard

It has no cholesterol. Packed with Vitamin A and Vitamin C. Also, rich in potassium and sodium.

117. Red-Lentil Hummus Sandwich

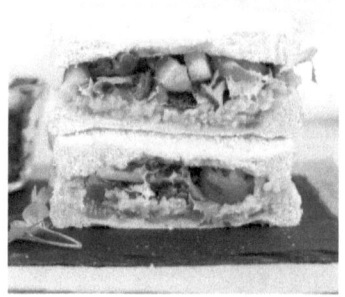

Lentils are an excellent alternative of chickpeas when it comes to making hummus. Making use of the red lentils in this recipe can be a good change of pace and you won't lose any of the metabolism-boosting advantages coupled with traditional hummus. You can also enjoy this dish with toasted whole-grain pita wedges or raw broccoli.

Ingredients

- One 1/2 tablespoons minced parsley
- Pinch sweet paprika

- One tablespoon extra-virgin olive oil for drizzling
- 1/4 teaspoon coriander
- One teaspoon red-wine vinegar
- Juice of 1/2 lemon
- Three tablespoons olive oil
- 1/2 smashed garlic clove
- 1/4 cup tahini
- 1/2 teaspoon sea salt for finishing
- One cup of cleaned red lentils
- Greek yogurt, optional

Method

1. Put lentils in a Two-quart pot; cover with two cups of water. Boil it and then reduce the heat and cook until it gets tender. Add coriander, vinegar, lemon juice, olive oil, garlic, tahini, salt and lentils in a food processor and blend until getting smooth.

2. To serve the dish spoon hummus into a shallow bowl. Sprinkle with parsley, paprika and olive oil. If you wish you can top it with Greek yogurt.

Facts to know

Lentils are loaded with protein and filling fiber, so you can go a long way keeping full. Moreover, it tastes great too.

118. Banana Nut Oatmeal

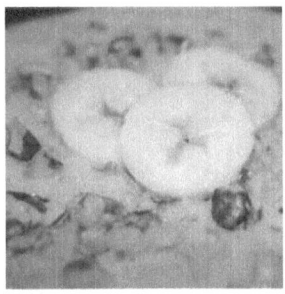

For sure, banana nut muffins are luscious; however, they're also a debacle for your waistline. So, with this recipe you can have one of the best alternatives of your morning meal with the savor you love with more fat-burning ingredients and fewer calories.

Ingredients

- One teaspoon ground cinnamon
- One tablespoon chopped walnuts
- One sliced banana
- One cup of water
- 1/2 cup of old-fashioned rolled oats

Method

1. Mix one cup of water and oats in a small microwave-safe bowl. Keep the microwave on at high for three minutes. Top with cinnamon, walnuts and banana slices.

Facts to know

Both banana and oatmeal are powerhouses for hunger-suppressing resistant starch which can get you halfway to your goal of 10 grams daily. Moreover, the walnuts supply the heart-healthy fats and can add some omega-3s for extra fat burning.

119. Greek Lentil Soup with Toasted Pita

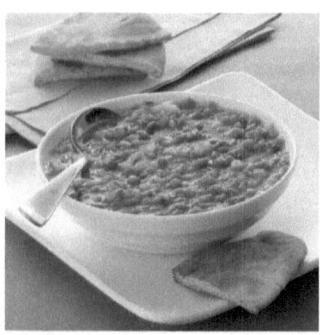

This thick Thirty-minute Greek soup with whole-grain pita wedges will help you to go on full until your next meal. The dish is packed with filling lentils, which provide more than half of the recommended intake of protein. In addition, per bowl you will get 5.3 grams of resistant starch.

Ingredients

- Four whole-grain pitas, each is toasted and cut into 4 triangles
- Two tablespoons fresh lemon juice (about 1 lemon)
- One cup of dry lentils

- Eight cups of water
- 1/2 teaspoon pepper
- 1/2 teaspoon salt
- Two teaspoons dried oregano
- Two minced garlic cloves
- One onion
- Two carrots, chopped and peeled
- Two chopped celery stalks
- One tablespoon olive oil

Method

1. Warm oil in a big Dutch oven over a medium heat. Add pepper, salt, oregano, garlic, onion, carrot and celery; cook for five minutes. Add the lentils and water. Boil for fifteen minutes. With a potato masher or hand blender, pulverize the soup until it gets semi-smooth and thick. Mix with lemon juice and serve with toasted pita triangles

Facts to know

Lentils are a grand source of fiber and resistant starch. If you wish you can double or triple this recipe and keep the leftovers in a freeze for individual servings.

120. Sunflower Lentil Spread

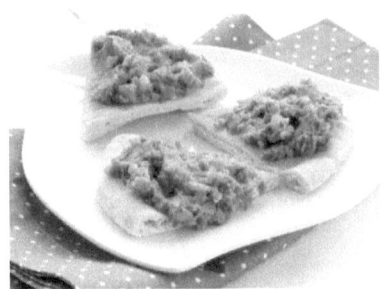

You can try this preparation on whole-grain pita wedges or in a veggie wrap for an afternoon snack. In both way, the mix of lentils and sunflower seeds will keep your belly satisfied.

Ingredients

- Two halved pitas
- Two tablespoons chopped fresh parsley

- One finely diced scallion
- One finely diced celery stalk
- Two tablespoons sunflower seeds
- 1/4 teaspoon pepper
- 1/4 teaspoon salt
- One tablespoon lemon juice
- One (15-ounce) can lentils, cleaned and drained

Method

1. Mix pepper, salt, lemon juice and lentils in a blender; blend it until getting smooth. Add parsley, scallions, celery and sunflower seeds. Microwave pita at HIGH for one minute. Finally, serve with spread.

Facts to know

As mentioned earlier lentils are a great source of resistant starch, and in this recipe, they will help you getting almost one-third of your way to your everyday 10-gram goal.

121. Vegan Caprese Salad

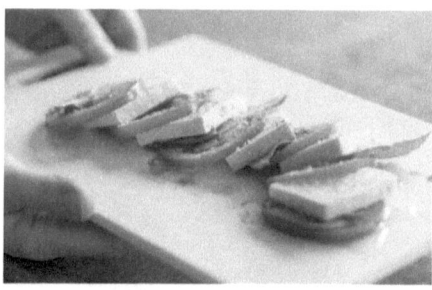

A beautiful vegan recipe, this one uses basil for the Italian twist to this classic recipe.

Ingredients

- 1 Medium Tomato
- 1/2 Avocado
- 6-8 Leaves Fresh Basil
- 1-2 Tsp. Extra Virgin Olive Oil
- 2 Tsp. Balsamic Vinegar
- Sea Salt & Pepper to Taste

Method

1. Arrange the fruit and veggie onto a plate. Top with the rest of the ingredients and enjoy!

Basil and its Health Benefits

Packed with vitamins and minerals. Basil has no cholesterol which makes it great for the heart. This ingredient has no carbohydrate.

122. Spiced Banana-Almond Smoothie

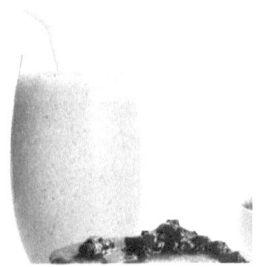

This satisfying smoothie is the just right post-workout snack to make you cool and can relieve your muscles aching. With protein-rich bananas and almonds which are loaded with resistant starch, you can have twofold of the appetite-suppressing ingredients.

Ingredients

- Two ice cubes
- One tablespoon honey
- 1/2 teaspoon ground cardamom
- One tablespoon almond butter
- One cup unsweetened almond milk
- One ripe banana

Method

1. Take all the ingredients in a blender and blend it until getting smooth.

Facts to know

This smoothie has low saturated fat and low cholesterol and can keep you happy as a breakfast or snack beverage.

123. Rice and Egg Salad-to-Go

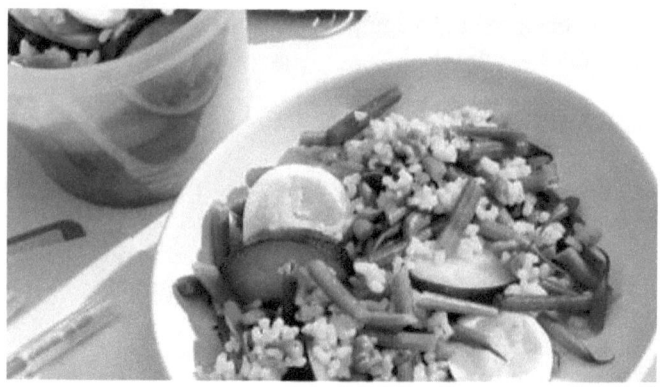

This Ten-minute salad-to-go mingles fresh flavors and colors from green beans, brown rice, walnuts, plums and a hard-boiled egg
Ingredients

Ingredients

- 1/2 cup cooked brown rice
- 1 cup cooked green beans, roughly chopped (3 oz.)
- 1 ripe plum, thinly sliced (3 oz.)
- 2 tablespoons (1/2 oz.) chopped walnuts
- 1 hard-cooked egg, sliced
- 1 teaspoon sesame oil
- 2 tablespoons fresh lime juice
- 1/4 teaspoon kosher salt
- Freshly ground black pepper, to taste

Method

1. Take the boiled egg, walnuts, plum, beans, and rice together in a portable container. Drizzle with pepper, salt, lime juice and sesame oil; toss gently to mix well. The dish is ready and you can refrigerate it up to two days.

Facts to know

Brown rice is a fiber-packed and hearty grain which is high in resistant starch and low in calories. A protein-packed walnuts and hard-boiled egg include healthy omega-3 fats and together they can help to keep you full.

124. All-American Chili

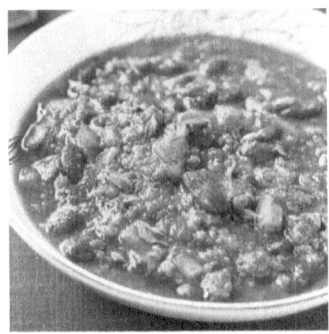

This recipe has two killer fat-burning ingredients: chili powder and red kidney beans. The kidney beans are full of protein and per serving can provide about thirty grams of that.

Ingredients

- 1/2 cup (two ounces) of frayed and reduced-fat sharp cheddar cheese
- Two (15-ounce) cans of drained no-salt-added kidney beans
- Two (28-ounce) cans no-salt-added whole tomatoes, coarsely chopped and un drained
- 1/4 cups of Merlot or other fruity red wine
- Two bay leaves
- 1/4 teaspoon salt
- 1/2 teaspoon freshly ground black pepper
- One teaspoon dried oregano
- Three tablespoons tomato paste
- One tablespoon ground cumin
- Two tablespoons brown sugar
- Two tablespoons chili powder
- One chopped jalapeño pepper
- One-pound ground sirloin
- Eight minced garlic cloves
- One cup of chopped green bell pepper
- Two cups of chopped onion
- Six ounces of hot turkey Italian sausage

Method

1. Warm a large Dutch oven over a medium to high heat. Take out the casings from sausage. Add sausage, green bell pepper, garlic cloves,

sirloin, jalapeño and onion. Cook for eight minutes or until the sausage get browned.

2. Add bay leaves, salt, black pepper, oregano, tomato paste, cumin, brown sugar, chili powder and cook for one minute. Put kidney beans, tomatoes and wine. Cook for one hour with a low heat with a cover over the oven. Shake it with a spoon occasionally. Uncover the oven and again cook for thirty minutes. Throw away the bay leaves. Finally, sprinkle each serving with cheddar cheese.

Facts to know

The chili powder contains a blazing compound known as capsaicin which can factually heat up your body and help you to burn more calories.

125. Strawberry Cauliflower Salad Delight

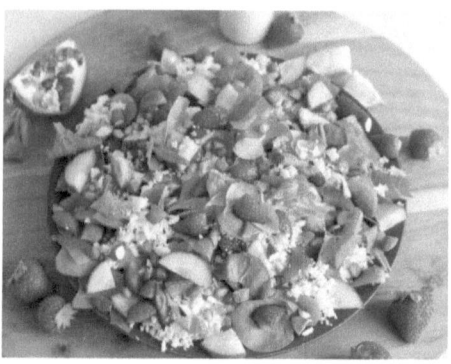

Made with wholesome strawberries and cauliflower, this delicious raw recipe is colorful, appetizing, easy to make and filling.

Ingredients

- 6 cups romaine lettuce, chopped
- 2 cups sliced strawberries
- 1 1/2 cups chopped cauliflower
- 1 small white onion
- A pinch of oregano
- A pinch of basil
- Salt and pepper to taste
- 1 teaspoon chopped garlic
- 1 teaspoon vinegar

Method

1. Arrange the salad in a plate. Just before serving add all the remaining ingredients to the salad and toss. Garnish with mint leaves and serve.

Little Red Strawberries for all the Healthy Reasons

Strawberries improve blood flow in the body and promote healthy growth. They are high in vitamins and minerals! Since strawberries have almost zero saturated fats, they are highly recommended to those looking to lose weight.

126. Creamy Cauliflower Salad with Ranch

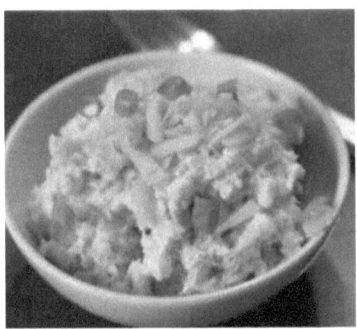

Another recipe made with raw cauliflowers. This one is a great variation to the boring raw food lovers. The ranch dressing used with the sour cream adds a unique flavor to the recipe.

Ingredients

- 2 large heads of Cauliflower = roughly 6 to 7 cups of florets
- 3 tbsps. Lemon Juice
- 3 Tbsps. Grape seed Oil
- 1/2 tsp Salt
- Pepper to Taste
- 2 Cups ripe cherry tomatoes
- Ranch Dressing
- Sour cream

Method

1. Arrange the cauliflowers in a bowl. Just before serving add the rest of the ingredients and toss. You are done!

The Amazing Cauliflower

Cauliflowers have zero cholesterol and trans fats which makes them an ideal choice for those looking to lose some extra pounds. They are very good for the eyes as they have rich in Vitamin A. Cauliflowers are also a great source of fiber.

127. Salad made with Shredded Brussels Sprouts

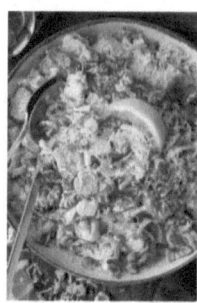

The raisins add the perfect sweetness to the Brussels sprouts. Packed with health, this amazing recipe is made with sunflower seeds and lemon for a slight tangy amazingness.

Ingredients

- 1 C. Brussels Sprouts, thinly sliced
- 1-2 Tbs. Raisins
- 1-2 Tbs. Roasted, Lightly Salted Sunflower Seeds
- Juice of 1/2 a Lemon
- 1/2 Tbs. Olive Oil
- 1/2 Tbs. Maple Syrup

Method

1. Add all the ingredients to the Brussels sprouts and enjoy. Garnish with parsley if you want to improve on the presentation.

Brussels Sprouts for the Health Conscious

Brussels sprouts are very rich in vitamin C and they are great for the skin. Brussels sprouts are also a good source of iron. Fiber in the Brussels sprouts makes them great for weight loss.

128. Brussels Sprouts with Chili Flakes and Pumpkin Seeds Topping

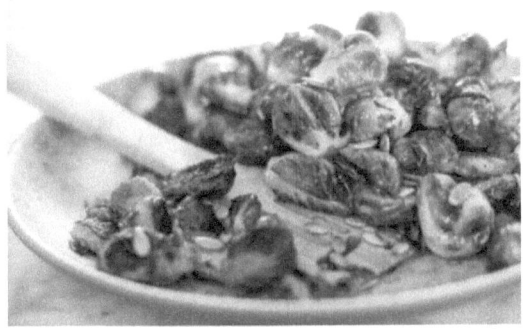

Another recipe made with the delightful Brussels sprouts, this delicious raw food recipe will take you by surprise with its unique texture and taste. The chili flakes and lime adds the required spice and tanginess to the recipe.

Ingredients

- 16 oz. Brussels sprouts, washed and ends trimmed
- ½ cup pumpkin seeds
- 1/2 cup cashews
- 2 tablespoons tamari
- 1/2 teaspoon smoked paprika
- 1 teaspoon chili powder
- 1 1/2 tablespoons lime juice
- 1 tablespoon olive oil
- 1/4 cup nutritional yeast

Method

1. Add the ingredients in a food processor and pulse. Dehydrate and store in an air tight container for two weeks. Enjoy!

Pumpkin Seeds and Health

Very good for losing weight as they are very high in fiber. Pumpkin seeds have zero cholesterol! Pumpkin seeds are an excellent source of magnesium in the body.

129. Raw Pesto Pasta with Pine Nuts and Carrots

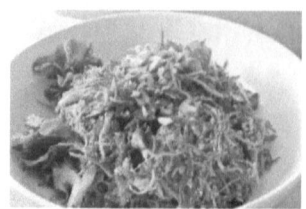

A classic raw twist to the traditional pasta, this vegan recipe is perfectly filling for your belly.

Ingredients

- 2 medium zucchinis
- 2 medium carrots
- 1 cup pine nuts
- 1/2 cup raw pumpkin seeds
- 2/3 cup Extra Virgin Olive Oil
- 1 cup fresh basil, stems included, packed tightly
- 1/2 teaspoon sea salt
- 1/2 garlic clove
- Black pepper to taste

Method

1. Shred your carrots and zucchini and set aside. Pulse all the other ingredients in a food processor. Serve together and enjoy!

The Benefits of Using Olive Oil

Excellent source of omega 3 and good fats, olive oil is very good for the eyes. For those losing weight, it is highly recommended that you substitute your regular oil with olive oil.

130. Tangy Kale Pesto

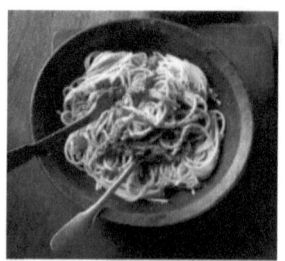

This recipe is made with kale and plenty of lemon for a lemony flavor. Tangy kale pesto is ideal for use as a spread on flax crackers.

Ingredients

- 1 bunch kale
- 1/4 cup nutritional Yeast
- 3/4 cup pecans
- ½ teaspoon sea salt
- zest of 1/2 lemon
- 1 tablespoon lemon juice, freshly squeezed
- 1 clove garlic, grated
- ¼ cup olive oil

Method

1. Remove stems from the bunch of kale. Include all the other ingredients in a food processor. Gradually add olive oil, until all the ingredients form a nice mixture. Spread on flax crackers and enjoy!

Health Benefits of Kale

This leafy green is an excellent source of vitamin A which makes it great for the eyes. Kale is also very rich in Vitamin C and B-6 which makes it very good for the skin and nails. Also, a very good source of potassium.

131. Kelp Noodles with Pesto Pasta

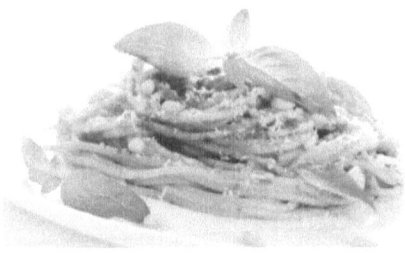

You will never be tired of this energizing recipe. You can also use the pesto recipe separately and use it as a salad dressing.

Ingredients

- 1 cup basil, parsley, arugula, kale
- 1 tsp. lemon juice or to taste

- 3-5 cloves garlic
- 1 Tbs. mellow white miso paste (cheesy taste)
- 1/2 tsp. Himalayan salt crystals
- 1/4 cup olive oil
- 1/2 cup pine nuts
- 1 pack of kelp noodles

Method

1. Toss the ingredients in a food processor and pulse. Make sure you don't totally liquefy the ingredients; some texture is good. Serve over the kelp noodles. Have fun eating!

Kelp is good for you!

This underwater plant is great for weight loss! It is packed with vitamins and minerals that help your body shed those extra pounds. Very rich in sodium which helps in maintaining the fluids in the body.

132. Spinach Basil Pesto with Raw Noodles

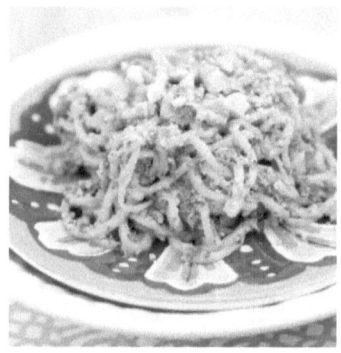

Lower in fat when compared to other pesto, this one is made with spinach and tomatoes.

Ingredients

- 2 1/2 cups packed spinach
- 3/4 cup fresh basil leaves
- 1/3 cup sun dried tomatoes, chopped
- 3 Tablespoons hemp seeds
- 3 Tablespoons lemon juice
- 2-3 Tablespoons water

- 3 Tablespoons olive oil
- 1 Tablespoon nutritional yeast
- 1 large clove garlic
- 1/2 teaspoon Himalayan salt
- Zucchini Noodles

Method

1. Toss all the ingredients in a food processor and form a nice mixture. Serve over zucchini noodles and enjoy! Improve presentation with some red chopped tomatoes.

Nutritional Value of Hemp Seeds

Hemp seeds have no saturated fats and Trans fats. Hemp seeds are also rich in fiber and protein. A great source of iron in the body.

133. Ravioli Made with Beets and Served with Pesto Oil

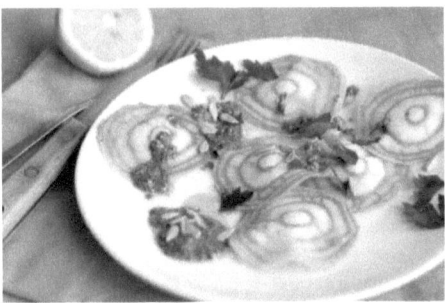

Sprinkled with pesto oil, this raw twist to the traditional ravioli is delicious and healthy.

Ingredients

- 3 – 4 large beetroots
- Juice of ½ lemon
- 1 ½ Tbsp. extra virgin olive oil
- Sea salt
- Pine Nut "Cheese"
- Pesto Oil
- Extra virgin olive oil
- Chives for garnish

Method

1. Thinly slice beets after peeling them. Place pine nuts cheese in between the beet roots (See the next recipe on how to make pine nuts cheese). Drizzle with pesto oil.

Lemony Lemons for all the Healthy Reasons

An excellent source of Vitamin C, lemons promote healthy skin and nails. Lemons help improve metabolism and subsequently trigger weight loss. Did you know lemons also have exceptional uses in the household cleaning chores?

134. Pine Nuts Cheese

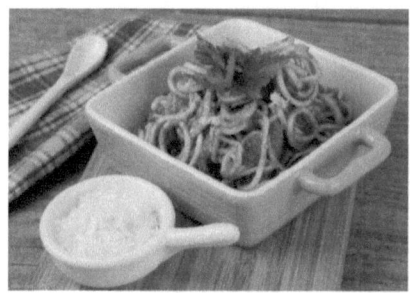

Made with pine nuts, this exceptional raw cheese recipe will taste good with anything!

Ingredients

- 1 cup pine nuts, soaked
- 1 Tbsp. minced shallot
- 2 Tbsp. minced chives
- 2 tsp. Nutritional yeast
- Zest of one lemon
- 2 Tbsp. lemon juice
- 1 Tbsp. extra virgin olive oil
- A couple pinches of smoked salt, to taste

Method

1. Soak and drain pine nuts for one hour. Blend all the ingredients together in a food processor. Enjoy your vegan cheese!

Wholesome Pine Nuts-Health Benefits

Pine nuts have zero cholesterol which makes it good for the heart. They are also rich in dietary fibers and help you stay full longer. Rich in Vitamin A and it is very good for the eyes.

135. Avocado Pesto with Parsley

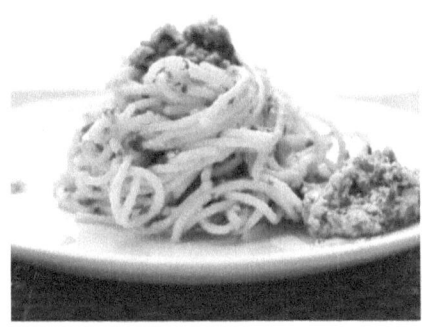

This avocado variation of pesto is made with parsley and uses lemon for its tangy bitterness and taste.

Ingredients

- One bunch of flat leaf parsley
- One avocado
- Two or three cloves of garlic
- The juice of one lemon
- A quarter cup of raw sunflower seeds
- Himalayan salt to taste

Method

1. Make a nice mixture of all the ingredients in a food processor. Add some Himalayan salt to you taste and enjoy!

Avocado for All Its Positive Health Effects

Avocados are great for a healthy heart as they have zero cholesterol! Because they are rich in fiber, avocados help you stay fuller, longer. They are also rich in minerals and vitamins!

136. Kale and Avocado Salad with Raw Black Olives

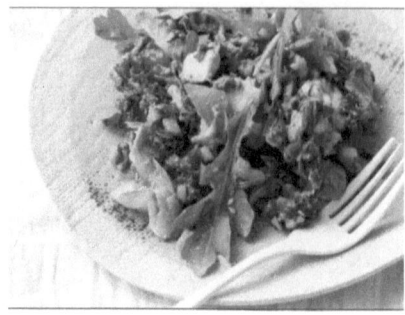

Olives give this kale and avocado salad a very different taste and color. A great variation and a must try for all the vegan lovers. The lime adds the tanginess to this delightful recipe!

Ingredients

- 1 Head of Kale
- ¼ Tsp. Salt
- 1 Lemon, squeezed
- 1 Tomato, chopped
- ½ Carrot, chopped
- ½ Avocado
- ¼ C. Black Olives
- ¼ C. Fresh Dulse
- Handful of Sprouts
- Handful of Goji Berries
- Handful of Fresh Herbs
- Handful of Raw Cashews

Method

1. Roughly chop all the ingredients and place in a bowl. Serve with black olives.

The Nutritious Goji Berries!

They have ZERO fat, so if you looking to lose weight, look for goji berries. They are a great source of iron and sodium. Goji berries also have zinc and calcium and they are very good for the bones.

137. Walnut, Celery and Apple Salad with Kale

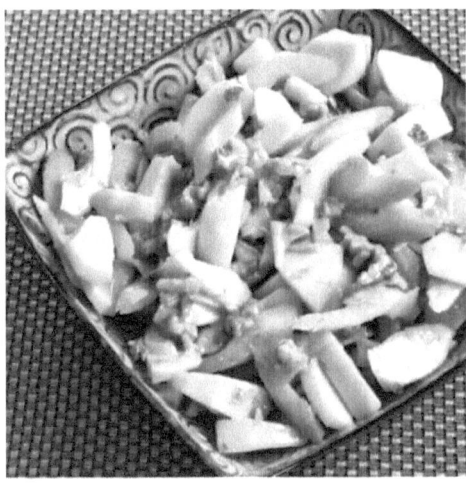

Apples give the recipe the sweetness it needs and walnuts add the crunch to this amazing salad made with celery and kale.

Ingredients

- 3-4 big kale leaves, chopped finely
- 2 Tbsp. lemon juice
- 1 medium apple, cored and diced
- 1 big celery rib, chopped
- handful of walnuts
- 1 Tbsp. good olive oil
- 1 Tbsp. good walnut oil
- ½ tsp balsamic vinegar
- Seasoning, to taste
- Top with sesame seeds

Method

1. Toss in the ingredients and mix them well before serving. Garnish with cilantro and enjoy!

Apples

A great source of iron and minerals! It helps fight bacteria in the body. A great antioxidant!

138. Mango Salad with Peaches and Lemon

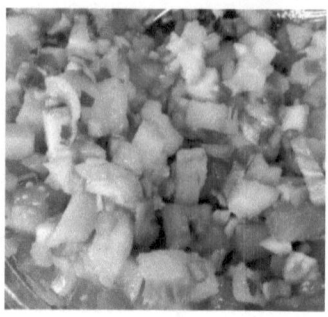

A very simple salad made with seasonal fruits and lemon.

Ingredients

- 1 peeled and diced Mango
- 1 peach, diced
- Juice of 1/4th lemon

Method

1. Arrange the fruits and squeeze a lemon in top. Enjoy!

Mangoes for the Season

Mangoes have NO fat! They are a great source of instant energy. Mangoes are also a good source of dietary fibers.

139. Grapes and Melon Salad

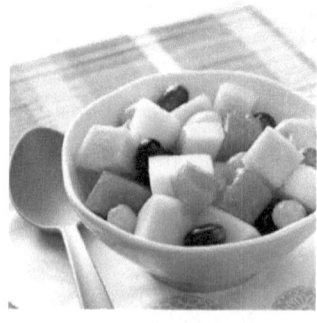

This is another simple fruit salad made with melon, grapes and orange juice.

Ingredients

- A bunch of grapes
- Half a melon, diced
- Juice of half an orange

Method

1. Arrange the fruit salad and squeeze in the orange juice. You are done!

The Seasonal Grapes

A great source of vitamin C. Also, rich in iron. Grapes also have no fat!

140. Raw Tuna Salad Recipe

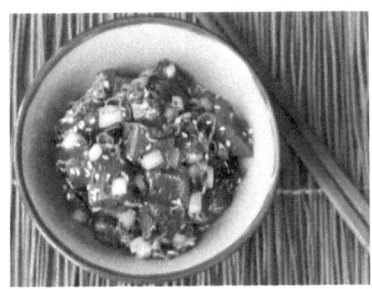

With the freshness of tuna, this simple tuna salad is a perfect lunch/dinner recipe. The sea salt used in the recipes adds an extra flavor to the recipe.

Ingredients

- 2 cups soaked sunflower seeds
- 1 tablespoon dulse
- 1 clove garlic
- 1 teaspoon lemon juice
- 1 teaspoon apple cider vinegar
- 1 teaspoon thyme
- 1/2 teaspoon sea salt

Method

1. Process all the ingredients in a food processor. Sprinkle with parsley and pickles and serve!

Tuna-Healthy for you!

Tuna is a great source of Omega 3. It is rich in good fats!

141. Basil and Cucumber Salad

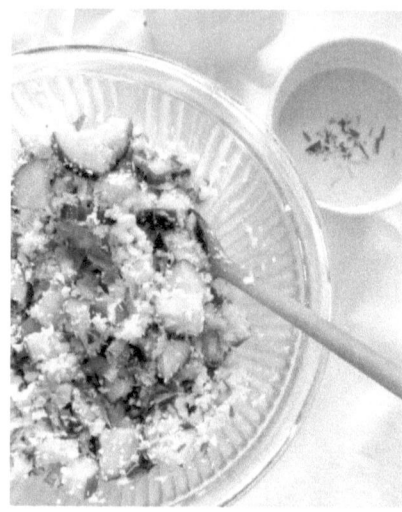

Made with refreshing cucumbers and lemon, this is a great salad with an Italian twist!

Ingredients

- 1 cucumber, quartered
- 1/3 head of cauliflower, chopped
- 1/2 of a red onion, diced small
- 1/4 cup fresh basil, chopped
- Juice of one lemon

Method

1. Arrange the salad on a plate and squeeze a lemon. Garnish with cilantro!

The Refreshing Cucumbers

Did you know 90% of the cucumber is water? Cucumbers are very good for the skin. It also helps improve complexion.

142. Apple and Apricot Salad with Ginger Dressing and Walnuts

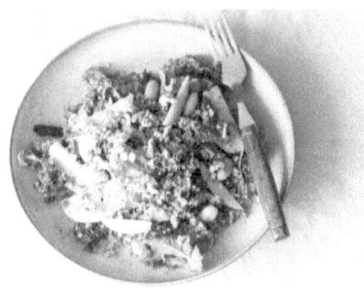

A perfect combination of tangy and sweet, this is a great raw food recipe made with fruits and kale.

Ingredients

- 1 head purple kale, chopped
- 6 dried apricots, sliced thinly
- 1/3 cup walnuts, raw
- 1 apple, sliced thinly
- Ginger dressing

Method

1. Toss in all the ingredients in a bowl. Top with ginger dressing.

Gingerly Ginger for the Healthy

Rich in Vitamin A. A good source of calcium and iron! No Trans fats.

143. Red Cabbage Salad

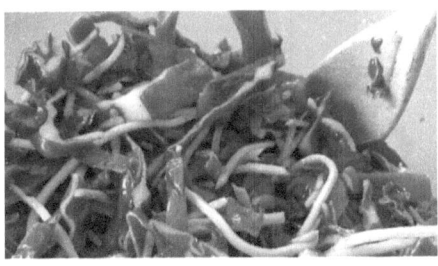

With a unique color, this recipe is both healthy and wholesome.

Ingredients

- 1/2 bunch curly kale, destemmed, washed, and finely chopped
- 1/2 cup carrot and red cabbage, thinly sliced
- 1/3 cup sauerkraut
- Single serving dulse
- 1/2 small avocado
- 2 tbsp. tahini
- 1 tbsp. lemon juice
- 1 tbsp. water
- 1/4 tsp powdered ginger

Method

1. Toss in all the ingredients together. You are done!

Cabbage with all its Health Benefits!

Excellent source of folate and vitamin C. A great source of potassium. Very low in calories.

144. Sugar Snap Pea Salad

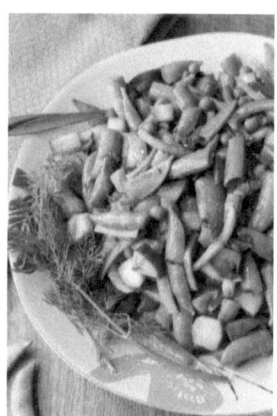

This colorful snap pea salad is made with cabbage and sesame seeds.

Ingredients

- 4 cups sugar snap peas, washed
- 1 3/4 cup shredded cabbage
- 1 scant tsp sesame oil

- 2 tbsps. rice wine vinegar
- 2 tsps. Tamari
- 1 cup sesame seeds
- Salt

Method

1. Toss in all the ingredients together. Use tomatoes for garnishing. Ta da! Done!

Sugar Snap Peas

It has NO fat or Trans-fat. A good source of dietary fiber. Also has protein.

145. Crunchy Green Apple and Red Cabbage Salad

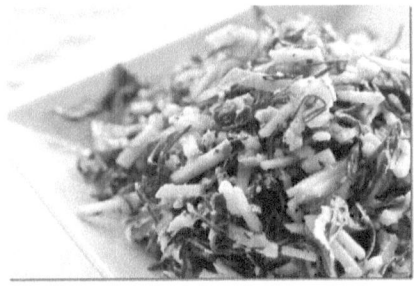

This easy colorful, easy recipe is an excellent choice for the health conscious!

Ingredients

- 3 cups thinly shredded red cabbage
- 1 large granny smith apple, shredded
- 2 tbsps. hemp seeds
- 1/4 cup tahini
- 3 tablespoons water
- 2 teaspoons maple syrup
- 1/2 teaspoon sesame oil
- Sea salt (to taste)
- 1 tablespoon apple cider vinegar

Method

1. Just add together all the ingredients in a bowl. Munch away!

Sesame Oil for the Health Conscious

It has no trans-fat. No carbohydrates. Has good fat!

146. Rainbow Salad with Coconut Oil

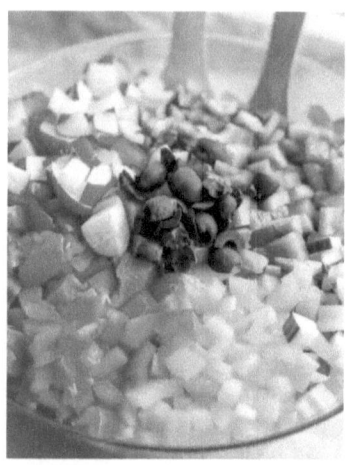

A wonderful mixture of crunchy and refreshing veggies, sprinkled with coconut oil.

Ingredients

- 3 Romaine Lettuce
- 1 small head Radicchio
- 1 large Carrot, peeled
- 1/2 Cucumber
- 1 Red Pepper
- 2 tbsp. Coconut Oil, melted
- 1 tsp. Lemon juice

Method

1. Arrange all the veggies on a platter. Sprinkle coconut oil and lemon juice. Voila, you're done!

Coconut Oil

Promotes healthy hair. Good source of minerals and vitamins. It boosts metabolism and boosts metabolism, which is why it helps in weight reduction.

147. Fiesta Carrot Salad

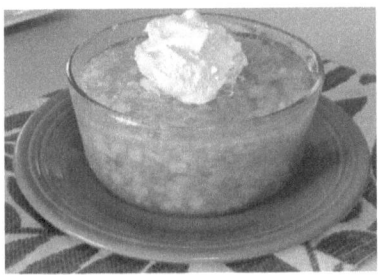

Another crunchy salad made with the delightful carrots!

Ingredients

- 8 medium carrots, sliced
- 1 bunch scallions, sliced
- 1 cup cherry tomatoes, halved
- 1 large avocado, diced
- Juice of one lemon
- 1 tbsp. olive oil

Method

1. Incorporate all the ingredients together. Squeeze in some lime and serve. Munch away!

Tomatoes and Health

Good source of dietary fiber. It has NO fat. Excellent source of vitamin A and C and they are very good for the eyes.

148. Walnut Salad with Guacamole Dressing

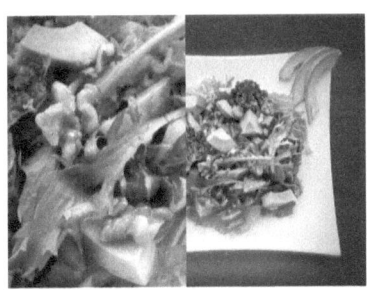

With all the health benefits of walnut, this recipe uses honey and garlic powder for the perfect Guacamole Dressing.

Ingredients

- 1/2 cup raw walnuts
- 1 head of green cabbage chopped
- 3-4 Avocados, mashed or diced
- 3 Tsp. fresh minced garlic or garlic powder
- 1/8 tsp. chipotle powder
- 1 tbsp. of raw honey or agave nectar
- 1/2 tbsp. pink Himalayan salt

Method

1. Add in all the ingredients together and toss right before serving. Enjoy!

Honey and its Benefits!

It is a great anti-oxidant. Provides instant energy. Packed with nutrients.

149. Raw Vegan Version of Waldorf Salad

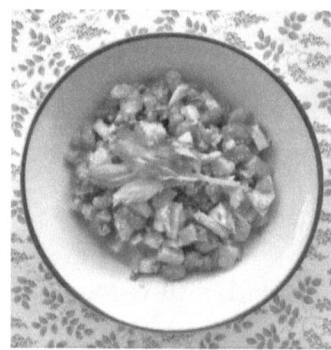

A perfect appetizer, this raw vegan version of the classic Waldorf salad uses cashews and honey instead of the mayo dressing!

Ingredients

- 1 bunch red kale, de-stemmed and finely chopped
- 4-5 large red apples, de-stemmed and chopped
- 5-6 celery stalks, chopped

- 1/2 cup walnut halves, chopped
- 1/2 cup Thompson raisins, soaked in warm water for 30 minutes
- Handful of Cashews
- 2 tbsps. Honey
- Salt to taste

Method

1. Incorporate all the ingredients together. Blend cashews, honey and salt together for a perfect vegan dressing. Enjoy!

Cashew

Did you know cashews have anti-depressant qualities? Cashews are packed with vitamins and good fats. They are very filling to the stomach.

150. Costa Rican Tomato Salad with Lime

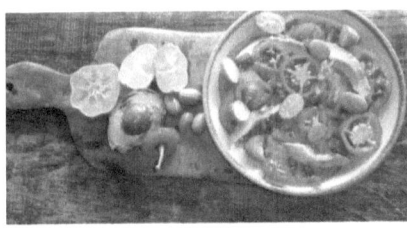

A light and healthy salad, perfectly made with cut up tomatoes, avocado and sweet pepper.

Ingredients

- 1/2 mandarin lime
- 1 big tomato (ripe)
- 3 small cherry tomatoes, halved
- 1 small sweet pepper
- 1/2 large avocado, sliced lengthwise
- 3 tbsps. fresh cilantro, finely chopped
- 5 wild cucumbers, halved or 1/2 small regular cucumber

Method

1. Arrange the cut-up fruits and veggies on a platter. Squeeze the mandarin lime on top. Bon appetite!

Sweet pepper and its health benefits

Rich in sodium. A good source of Vitamins, especially Vitamin A. It also has iron.

151. Watermelon and Peach Salad with Lime

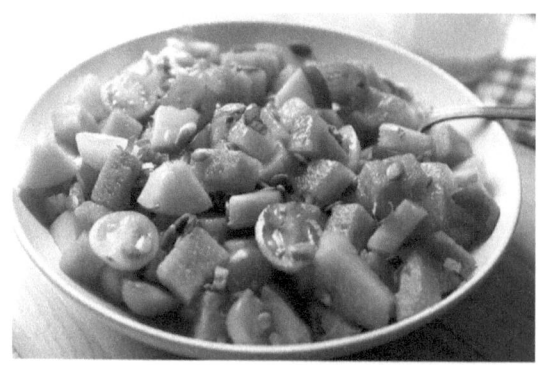

A delicious salad made with watermelons and peaches.

Ingredients

- 4 cups seedless watermelon, cubed
- 1 cup tomatoes, diced the same size as watermelon pieces
- 2 peaches, sliced 1/4 inch thick
- Juice of 2 limes
- 1 tsp coconut nectar (or raw honey or agave)
- Dash sea salt
- 1/4 cup extra virgin olive oil
- Handful basil, whole or chiffonade
- 1/4 cup pumpkin seeds (toasted or raw)

Method

1. Place the fruits in a large mixing bowl. Add the other ingredients for the dressing. Enjoy the scrumptiousness of your salad!

Watermelon and its deliciousness!

It has no cholesterol. Very rich in vitamin C. Also has iron!

152. Orange Salad with Avocado and Black Olives

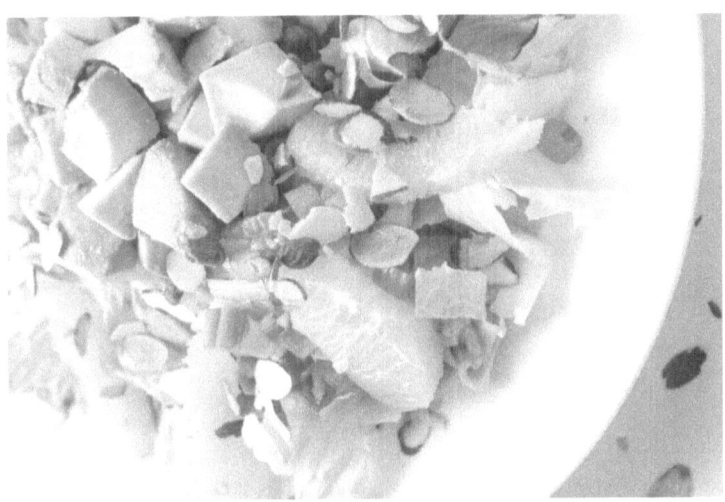

This is another fresh salad with all its freshness of oranges and mint leaves, combined with avocado for a unique texture and taste.

Ingredients

- 2-3 C Salad greens
- 1/2 Avocado, sliced
- 1 Orange, segmented
- 1/4 Red onion, minced
- 1 tbsp. Apple cider vinegar
- 1 tbsp. extra-virgin olive oil
- 1 tbsp. Minced black olives
- Salt & Pepper

Method

1. Incorporate the salad ingredients together. Enjoy the freshness of the oranges and the avocados. Garnish with mint leaves.

Red Onion

It is a great antioxidant. Good for the eyes! Lowers the risk of developing cancer and also reduces blood pressure.

153. Strawberry and Spinach Salad

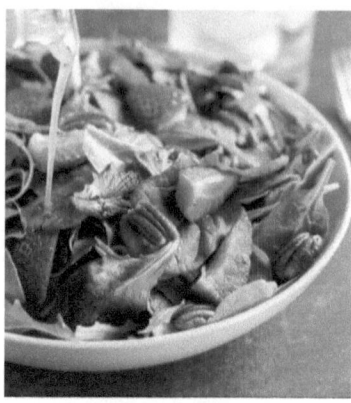

This recipe encompasses health and taste. Prepared with spinach, this recipe also used strawberries for its sweetness and health benefits.

Ingredients

- 1 bunch spinach
- 1/2 avocado, sliced
- 10 strawberries, sliced
- 2 chives, diced
- 1/4 cup roasted and halved hazelnuts
- 2 tbsps. sunflower seeds
- 2 tbsps. red wine vinegar
- 1 tbsp. lemon juice
- 1 Tsp agave nectar
- 1/2 tsp salt
- Freshly ground pepper
- 1/4 cup olive oil

Method

1. Don't forget to wash the spinach before you toss in all the ingredients together. Enjoy!

Spinach and Health!

A very good anti-oxidant, it helps protect the body from bacteria. Very good for the eyes. Excellent for weight loss.

Final Words

I would like to thank you for downloading my book and I hope I have been able to help you and educate you about something new.

If you have enjoyed this book and would like to share your positive thoughts, could you please take 30 seconds of your time to go back and give me a review on my Amazon book page!

I greatly appreciate seeing these reviews because it helps me share my hard work!

Again, thank you and I wish you all the best with your cooking journey!

Last Chance to Get YOUR Bonus!

FOR A LIMITED TIME ONLY – Get Olivia's best-selling book *"The #1 Cookbook: Over 170+ of the Most Popular Recipes Across 7 Different Cuisines!"* absolutely FREE!

Readers have absolutely loved this book because of the wide variety of recipes. It is highly recommended you check these recipes out and see what you can add to your home menu!

Once again, as a big thank-you for downloading this book, I'd like to offer it to you *100% FREE for a LIMITED TIME ONLY!*

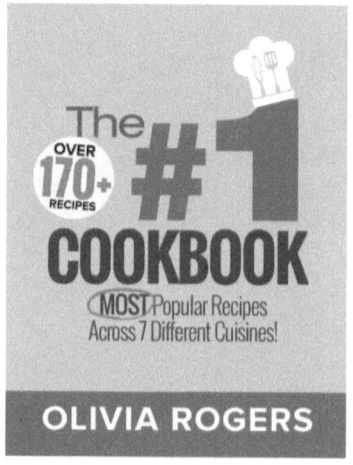

Get your free copy at:

TheMenuAtHome.com/Bonus

Disclaimer

This book and related site provides recipe and food advice in an informative and educational manner only, with information that is general in nature and that is not specific to you, the reader. The contents of this book and related site are intended to assist you and other readers in your personal efforts. Consult your physician or nutritionist regarding the applicability of any information provided in our information to you.

Nothing in this book should be construed as personal advice or diagnosis, and must not be used in this manner. The information provided about conditions is general in nature. This information does not cover all possible uses, actions, precautions, side-effects, or interactions of medicines, or medical procedures. The information in this site should not be considered as complete and does not cover all diseases, ailments, physical conditions, or their treatment.

No Warranties: The authors and publishers don't guarantee or warrant the quality, accuracy, completeness, timeliness, appropriateness or suitability of the information in this book, or of any product or services referenced by this site.

The information in this site is provided on an "as is" basis and the authors and publishers make no representations or warranties of any kind with respect to this information. This site may contain inaccuracies, typographical errors, or other errors.

Liability Disclaimer: The publishers, authors, and other parties involved in the creation, production, provision of information, or delivery of this site specifically disclaim any responsibility, and shall not be held liable for any damages, claims, injuries, losses, liabilities, costs, or obligations including any direct, indirect, special, incidental, or consequences damages (collectively known as "Damages") whatsoever and howsoever caused, arising out of, or in connection with the use or misuse of the site and the information contained within it, whether such Damages arise in contract, tort, negligence, equity, statute law, or by way of other legal theory.

www.ingramcontent.com/pod-product-compliance
Lightning Source LLC
Chambersburg PA
CBHW030000110526
44587CB00011BA/927